the INsid

Volume 2

the INside effects
Volume 2

How the Body Heals Itself

Featuring:

Marcus Bird, Kelly Brogan, Kim D'Eramo, Bradley Nelson,
Amandha Vollmer, Alec Zeck, and Lisa Warner

— and —

Contributing Authors – Aisha Ahmed, Renita Brannan,
Stephanie Dobranski, Susan Green, Michele Griffith, Holly
Hallowell, Sophia Harvey, Bethany Miller, Kerstin Opitz,
John Stringer, and Ishita Todi

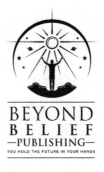

BEYOND
B E L I E F
—PUBLISHING—
YOU HOLD THE FUTURE IN YOUR HANDS

ISBN: 978-1-957972-05-3

This book was created in honor of all the doctors who have dedicated themselves to natural healing and all who are committed to healing themselves naturally.

Contents

Acknowledgments

It is with deep appreciation that I thank all the experts who said YES to participating in *the INside effects* film project: Darius Barazandeh, Marcus Bird, Kathleen Bobak, Lee Carroll, Kyle Cease, Deanna Courtney, Tom Cowan, John Demartini, Kim D'Eramo, Julie Renee Doering, Jeffrey Gignac, Mia Hohl, Karen Kan, Andrew Kaufman, Cathleen King, Erin Kinney, Matty Lansdown, MariaElena Marks, Rollin McCraty, Lynne McTaggart, Monika Muranyi, Bradley Nelson, Clint G. Rogers, Ken Rohla, JP Sears, Craig Shoemaker, Amandha Vollmer, Lisa Warner, and Mikki Willis.

Thank you to Erik Arthur Peterson, Theo Hall, Jordan Craig, Brian Dillon, Gabriel Valda, Callum Shallenberger, Mikal Masters, Nevaeh Pillsbury, Cruz Christian Carriere, Drew Thomsen, Erik Van Yserloo, Bob Sima, Shannon Plummer, Trisha Schmalhofer, and Maura Leon S., for your participation during the filmmaking process and after.

Thanks to Bob Proctor, Jack Canfield, Adam Markel, Joe Vitale, Michael Beckwith, Rickie Byars, and John Demartini for being such great mentors and for always saying yes. Your support over the years has been instrumental in my success as an author, publisher, and now a filmmaker.

Thank you to our incredible team who brought this book forward to completion and to the world one step at a time: Maggie Mills, Heather Taylor, Bethany Knowles, Autumn Carlton, MaryDes, Nida Palpallatoc, and Rudy Milanovich.

Introduction

When we decided to start a publishing business twenty years ago, we were very clear about the authors we wanted to publish. Our mentors had taught us, "You are the five people you spend the most time with." We wanted to surround ourselves with successful cutting-edge difference makers. Because of this, the first fifty books we published were authored by functional medical doctors. Functional medical doctors are *medical professionals who specialize in finding the root causes of disease*. They work holistically, considering the full picture of your physical, emotional, mental, and sometimes even spiritual health — considering factors like diet, hormonal changes, genetics, prescription and over-the-counter medications, and other lifestyle choices.

We soon discovered that the people we wanted to serve the most were so busy being in service to others, they didn't have time to sit down and write a book themselves. They needed a book to share their mission, vision, and gifts, but had no time to write it. This led us to the creation of a process we call *The YouSpeakIt Book Program*. Our process allows these difference makers to come to seven phone calls, and in those seven calls we lead them through speaking their book. It brought ease and grace to the book creation process, and ultimately this process ended up being one of the things that set us apart from other publishers.

While working with these medical professionals and reading their books, we learned a lot about how the body has the ability to heal itself. Keith had an experience as a child when his aunt used non-traditional healing methods to dissolve cancer in two weeks. This implanted into his mind the thought and belief "the body has the ability to heal itself," which is why he decided that for his first full-feature film, he would produce and direct a documentary called *the INside effects: How the Body Heals Itself*. This film would allow him to really dive into the subject he has such a passion for. This film, and the doctors, scientists, and health advocates he interviewed, not only validated a lot of his beliefs, but also opened a new world of information he hadn't studied and researched.

Keith realized at one point during the film production process that he was only going to be able to interview a limited number of experts, and the questions he was asking each health advocate in the film covered three main topics. He thought to himself, *I want to provide people who have just watched the film with their next steps and introduce them to more experts*. This is where the idea for this book was born. Its focus is on one thing and one thing alone … now that you have learned the body does indeed have the ability to heal, how do you do it?

We have purposely asked all the experts the same three questions. This allows you to get specific answers regarding healing, while allowing you to feel into who the best teachers for you are. We suggest you reach out to those you feel most connected to, work with them, and hire them. If you've discovered this book without seeing the movie, we highly suggest you watch it (www.theINsideeffects.com), as the film is also created to introduce you to the top experts in their field. Reach out to them as well.

We trust this book will guide you to learning and discovering alternative methods for healing. It has been an absolute pleasure to interview the authors and provide this valuable information. Enjoy the read.

Warmly,

Keith and Maura Leon S.

www.BeyondBeliefPublishing.com

www.LeonSmithPublishing

www.YouSpeakItBooks.com

www.BabypiePublishing.com

Aisha Ahmed

WHEN AND HOW DID YOU FIRST DISCOVER THAT THE BODY HAS THE INNATE ABILITY TO HEAL ITSELF?

My discovery began in 2011 right after I gave birth to my first child. I had some complications and developed chronic back pain. Initially, I had no idea what was going on, so I started going from doctor to doctor — all sorts of specialists and nothing was helping. The pain stayed with me for five long years, and it badly impacted my quality of life. There were so many things I had tried by that point and nothing was helping.

Eventually, I was able to understand that because I had a lot of unprocessed grief from the loss of my father, it was stuck in my body and manifested as chronic back pain. My journey with this back pain led me to discover holistic healing modalities. I came across a beautiful book that was all about processing emotions, and I decided to give it a go.

What I learned was fascinating and amazing — our unprocessed emotions and traumas stay in our subconscious mind, holding a literal place in the cells of our body, and then they manifest as physical, mental, or emotional symptoms. I released the trapped emotions that were staying in my pelvis and womb because of the traumatic past experiences and unpleasant delivery events. When I woke up the next morning, I was literally pain-free.

It was surprising at first. I was expecting the pain to come back, but it never returned. That is when I made it my soul mission to help people release the unresolved, stuck energy from their body, and it opened up a whole new world for me.

The second major life shift for me was in 2018 when my daughter was diagnosed with *Tourette syndrome*. The doctors told us she just had to learn to live with it. I refused to accept that as a diagnosis and took matters into my own hands. I started uncovering all the missing pieces of why our body creates certain imbalances and symptoms and how the body has the ability to heal itself. All you have to do is make the conditions right for the body to heal.

I began working with my daughter by helping her remove the heavy metals from her body, focusing on healing her gut, removing all the emotional overload, and especially the inherited ancestral emotional baggage, along with a deep focus on healing myself and my husband, as we understood she was showing us what we needed to address within ourselves. We were able to reverse her condition one hundred percent within three weeks.

These two major events further confirmed that this is my soul mission — to help people heal by trusting their body's innate intelligence. We just have to make the environment right for the body to heal.

WHY DO YOU THINK IT'S SO IMPORTANT FOR PEOPLE TO BE AWARE OF HOW THE BODY HEALS ITSELF?

Our body's natural, innate healing system is embedded within us by design. Our subconscious mind takes care of millions of bodily functions daily without us having to be aware of it. For example, breathing, digestion, muscle function, scars getting healed — it is all happening all the time.

Unfortunately, big pharma brainwashes and programs our minds to only one way of healing. But as we know, stats show the allopathic system is the third largest cause of death in North America. It is based on suppression of symptoms and not finding the root cause. This is making more and more people sick. I see people giving their power away to big pharma because of the belief this is the only way to heal, and simultaneously they believe any alternative healing modality is woo woo, or a scam. Whereas, in reality, looking at all aspects of mind, body, and soul allows a person to heal holistically.

I am very focused on resetting these beliefs for people. The good thing is people are waking up, especially after what we saw happen following the COVID vaccinations, and studies are out in the open now. Most doctors do not emphasize the importance of food, stress management, or even the importance of getting proper sleep. When all these things are considered as part of the healing system, holistically helping somebody heal, there will be fewer people getting sick. A big part of it is also relieving the suppressed, unprocessed emotions and traumas—resetting belief systems and how you see life with all the thoughts from your own childhood experiences. Eliminating heavy metals and reducing stress make the conditions right for the body to heal.

WHAT ADVICE DO YOU HAVE FOR CREATING HEALTH AND VITALITY FROM THE INSIDE OUT?

We need to return to nature and simplify our lifestyle. We need to eliminate toxins, move our bodies, come back to eating natural healthy foods, and do the emotional processing. That may include getting help from a professional.

You do not have to eat the whole elephant all at once. Begin by making small life changes—moving your body, spending time in the sunshine, and getting in the habit of listening to your body's wisdom. Be mindful of what is inside because your outside environment is showing what you are harboring inside. Be mindful of your thoughts and what emotions ride you, and then make adjustments when you are not in harmony with yourself and with your true spirit. When you return to your spiritual center, what is your soul telling you, what is your body saying to you, what are your emotions telling you? These are all messengers giving us important information about where you are giving your power away and where you need to trust and strengthen your inner voice.

When we understand all the answers are within us, when we are one with nature and with our true nature, we let go of a lot of heavy conditioning, societal programming, and trauma. That is when we return to homeostasis and make the conditions right for expedient health and vitality from the inside out.

When focusing on healing the root cause of any symptoms, we must consider what emotions we are digesting. Are we letting go of the shame, resentment, hurt, and inner child unprocessed traumas? When we bring the inner environment in alignment and let go of the old stagnant beliefs we have around health and healing in our subconscious mind, then we create a beautiful, external reality that is healthy and vital.

About the Author

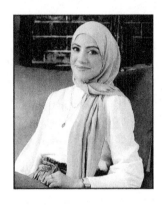

Aisha Ahmed is a Certified Subconscious Mind Expert and Quantum Energetics Healer, corporate trainer, and mentor for wellness business owners. She has impacted the lives of thousands of clients all over the world—from corporate CEOs to industry leaders in entrepreneurship, coaches, and media personalities. They have tried everything and lost hope in their healing. Aisha shows them how to take back their power and step into freedom and fulfilment, with her transformative one-on-one, group, and corporate healing programs.

With over seventeen years of extensive training around the globe with phenomenal spiritual teachers and healers and certification in the latest bioenergetic, quantum science, and neuroscience-based modalities,

Aisha's mission is to help people create successful heart-led legacy and impact through their business without compromising their joy, relationships, and especially time with their families.

Aisha resides in Canada with her husband, also a Subconscious Healing expert and co-facilitator of their global healing mission, along with their two children. She is the founder of Aisha Heals and has a very active and engaged community on Instagram where she gives lots of value and support to people.

Here's a free subconscious activation bundle designed to unlock your most abundant timeline by rewiring your subconscious mind: https://programs.aishaheals.com/book.

Aisha is most active with her community on Instagram, so follow her there for all her latest programs, free content, live healing sessions, and more at www.instagram.com/aishaheals, and you can check out her services on her website www.aishaheals.com.

Marcus Bird

WHEN AND HOW DID YOU FIRST DISCOVER THAT THE BODY HAS THE INNATE ABILITY TO HEAL ITSELF?

I went through a life-changing experience some twenty-five, thirty years ago when I gave myself chronic fatigue syndrome. At the time, I was very focused on standard western medicine and did not know a lot about anything else. When I became ill and decided to get sicker and sicker, I obviously went to the doctor. The doctor took a lot of blood tests and pretty much said, "There is nothing wrong with you," yet I kept getting sicker. I kept going to more and more doctors. They took more and more blood tests, and they always came back saying, "Nothing is wrong with you and if you just get a little more sleep, you will be fine."

I got to the point in my illness when I could no longer function as a normal human being, could not hold down a job, could not socialize with friends and family, and could not watch television or listen to the radio. I could not do anything except pretty much just lie in bed. That is when I realized something else had to be out there and I was not going to stay sick.

I started a beautiful internal and external search for something else. Through that search, I realized the body has the ability to heal itself. I then went on a journey of self-healing using the discoveries I found, and I healed more quickly from chronic fatigue than most people do.

WHY DO YOU THINK IT'S SO IMPORTANT FOR PEOPLE TO BE AWARE OF HOW THE BODY HEALS ITSELF?

It is important for people to be aware of the power and resources they have within themselves. Often when you do not have that understanding, you tend to give your power away to anybody who says they have a magic pill to heal you, which can cause even more disease. Apart from that, the options out there often destabilize other aspects of the body. It might heal or help with one aspect of the issue you are dealing with, but then it destabilizes other aspects of your body. You end up going round and round in circles. You fix one thing, then cause something else to go wrong. You fix that thing and cause another problem. It is a never-ending spiral of ease and dis-ease. When you realize you can connect into the deeper power within you, then you resolve the issues and the problems you are experiencing, and you embrace the power to curtail or fend off any other possibilities that might enter your field. It is an empowering experience to realize that you have all of the resources within you to stabilize yourself and heal yourself.

WHAT ADVICE DO YOU HAVE FOR CREATING HEALTH AND VITALITY FROM THE INSIDE OUT?

Explore. Be inquisitive. Reconnect to the part of you that has the answers and the ability to heal itself or at least support itself on the healing journey. Go on a journey of self-discovery to find out other things that can assist and support you to find the things which work specifically for you. For most diseases and illnesses, there are very specific things you need to do that may not be the same as what other people experience or find to be successful. You have to find your own pathway to better health, to restabilize yourself to wellness and vitality. If you can keep a really inquisitive mind, if you can spend time connecting with yourself, then when you start to look outside of yourself and start to research all of the amazing natural harmonic ways to heal and restabilize yourself, you become vital again. Then you will be able to connect to the things that are best for you, and which resonate the most with you. There could be a myriad of natural remedies and therapies and people and systems and processes that help you.

On my healing journey, the very first thing I did was start to meditate. I started to go within. I started to explore the inner realm of myself. Before then I went outside of myself to discover some of the amazing methodologies, people, natural healing, remedies, and processes that exist in the world. The very first step is to dive within and start exploring the inner realms of the self. Remain really inquisitive and interested in exploring all of the possible options. By doing this first, you reconnect with yourself, and then you can remain sensitive to what is in resonance with you, what is in harmony with you, what methodology, what healing, what remedies, what natural things are in resonance with you and are going to give you the ability to amplify the most beautiful well-stabilized, harmonic you.

About the Author

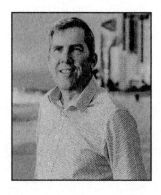

Marcus is a creator, channel, and coach. Some call him the Wellness Futurist or Dimensional Resonance Coach but really, he is a channel and global activator for full potential. Marcus is on a mission to move 1% of the population into a cosmic conscious state.

After a life-changing experience, Marcus was thrust into the world of channeling a higher dimensional being called AMEED. When Marcus gave himself chronic fatigue syndrome, little did he know it was to change his life completely — from corporate Jedi to channel, healer, and teacher of ancient information. As a researcher and channel of the sacred ancient Egyptian healing called *Aboukra*, sacred geometry, and modern quantum physics, Marcus began to teach about stabilizing people so they can step into and activate their full potential.

Marcus is here to support, help, and inspire you to achieve a better outcome, better life, and more success — whatever that is for you. He sees the potential in every human to step into the infinite possibility and be all you are here to be. "I REALLY want that for all humans as we step into a higher level of consciousness and Cosmic Consciousness."

To support you in deepening your healing journey and embracing the Inside Effects, please download this FREE Pyramid Meditation and join our Facebook Group, Heart of the Matrix.

https://www.dimensionalcoach.com/pyramidmeditation

https://www.facebook.com/groups/heartofthematrix

Renita Brannan

WHEN AND HOW DID YOU FIRST DISCOVER THAT THE BODY HAS THE INNATE ABILITY TO HEAL ITSELF?

About twenty years ago I realized how nutrition was having a significant impact on my son's health. He had been vomiting and coughing all night for months. When we eliminated dairy from his diet, the coughing completely subsided in a matter of a day or two. That is where it started, but not where it finished. That was my first glimpse at how the body can heal itself.

I spent time investigating how chemicals affect our bodies. I learned a lot about macronutrients, which are protein, fat, and carbohydrates; micronutrients, which are vitamins, minerals, and trace minerals; and phytonutrients, which are antioxidants that help reverse aging and reduce inflammation. I learned about the endocannabinoid system and that everybody should be nourishing it because it is super important for the overall health of the body; piezoelectricity, which is movement; and phototherapy, which is an asset that people need to learn about because it is so easy to tap into when beginning to heal their bodies. Then, of course, hydrotherapy.

God has had me on this adventure of macro, micro, phyto, endo, piezo, photo, and hydro. When you understand all of these elements and how they can restore and heal the body, it is miraculous what we have our hands on and how God designed our bodies to heal naturally with all these natural elements.

The biggest revelation I have had in the last few years is how light heals, and sun heals, and the different frequencies of light healing. About a year and a half ago, we went on an adventure with my dad's legs. We had been doctoring with all of the amazing modalities and treatments I know about, but nothing was healing his legs, which had been oozing and very swollen for about six months.

Then someone introduced me to phototherapy technology. I put a patch on his body. Within twenty-four hours all of the swelling had subsided. All the ooze we had seen for six consecutive months stopped. In that moment I realized, "Holy cow! Light heals." And what was in this patch doing this remarkable mechanism of healing my dad's legs? That is why I went down the path to phototherapy and is the path I am on right now because healing is all about frequency, sound, and light. Those modalities are what we are going to use to restore and heal our bodies.

Why do you think it's so important for people to be aware of how the body heals itself?

It is important for people to be aware of how the body heals itself because we all have the power to be well. The first step is to take back your power by believing you can. Believe the future can be better than the present, and then seek information. When you seek, you will find. Open your mind and your heart and your being and ask, "How can I be well, God? What can I do to be well?" Be prepared, because you are going to be in a flow you have never experienced before, where God reveals the healing modalities available to all of us.

For five decades, we have been inundated by the pharmaceutical world and have been trained we need a bio-chemical approach to healing—which is a pill for every ill. Now we realize, for example, with phototherapy, light affects the biochemistry of the body. When we go outside in the sunlight, it affects our hormones and all the healing mechanisms, such as activating peptides.

Peptides are naturally built-in healing strains of amino acids our bodies need. When we go outside in the sunlight and light hits our skin, our dermis, and eventually our epidermis, it activates a whole host of healing that optimizes our health—our skin health, our longevity, our sleep regulation, our mood, and so much more. Tapping into phototherapy and hydrotherapy, these incredible modalities of healing that are really upcoming, is going to be the future of healthcare. It is noninvasive, incredibly affordable, and amazingly effective.

WHAT ADVICE DO YOU HAVE FOR CREATING HEALTH AND VITALITY FROM THE INSIDE OUT?

I think everything is an inside job. It's like that old saying, "What comes first, the chicken or the egg?" What comes first—the healing or the belief? We begin by believing we can be well, and then we put our mind, our energy, our attention, and our heart in that focused energy source of asking, "What can I do to improve my quality of life? What can I do to be well?"

Then we must imagine we are already healed. "I am healed. I am whole. I am healthy." Believe God designed our bodies to heal. He did. Light is mentioned over two hundred fifty times in the Bible. In the very first verse of the Bible, God says, "Let There Be Light."

James 1:17 reads, *"Every good and perfect gift is from above, coming* down from the *Father* of the *heavenly lights,* who does not change like shifting shadows." Light is a healing gift. If you have ever been sick for a season or had a loved one, an aging parent, or a child who is sick, when you get well it is a gift from heaven. We all have that right in our hands, right now. It is accessible to every one of us if we want to access that innate ability of our body's healing mechanism. The first thing we have to do is believe and align the facts that we can be well and we are healing machines. I walk around my house and say out loud, "My body is a healing machine. My body is a healing machine." Doing that opens up my mind, my heart, and my energy to the flow of what is possible with healing.

The first stage is believing, and the next is seeking. When you do that, God will lead you to divine appointments where you step into modalities or alternative ways of healing or viewing something you have never seen before. It is available to all of us. Faith is effective in the healing process. Have the faith you can be well and move in that direction.

About the Author

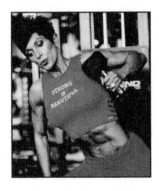

First and foremost, Renita Brannan is a child of God! She resides in North Dakota with her husband Scott, three sons (Beau, Truitt, and Rocco), and girl dog, Nike.

Renita has a Bachelor of Arts in Physical Education and Business from Dickinson State University, and she is a former TV personality for NBC affiliate KFYR TV as their Health and Fitness Expert.

Continued education and a passion for knowledge have been integral to Renita's success with over twenty-five years of accumulated credentials.

Renita has certifications in over thirty modalities of fitness, including:

Certified Nutrition Coach, International Board of Nutrition and Fitness Coaching; ACE Certified

Advanced Personal Trainer; ACE Lifestyle and Weight Management Consultant; ACE Group Fitness Instructor; FiTOUR Master Trainer; FitBeach: International Master Trainer; Sports Conditioning Specialist Certified Trainer; Senior Fitness Certified for Elderly Fitness; Master Trainer for Aqua Rock and "Delay the Disease" Certified for those with Parkinson's, neurodegeneration, and movement disorders; Certified Behavioral Change Specialist, Certified Biblical Health Coach, Certified Endocannabinoid System / CBD Physiology and Health Certified.

Renita was featured on CNN Headline News for Testimony Tuesday, helping the state of North Dakota lose 100,000 pounds.

She has co-authored two Amazon bestsellers, *Nice and Fat* and *My CBD Money-Tree*.

Renita created PFC Plate, the world's first nutritional blood sugar stabilization tool to help individuals rewire their brains through repetition and nourish their bodies with food. A clinical study showed 19.8 inches of body fat were lost in eight weeks. A study proved a statistically significant reduction in A1C. In addition, she just launched a PFC bar to aid in the process of health, vitality, and weight loss: www.pfcplate.com.

Renita has pioneered the CBD industry in North Dakota and across the U.S. by playing an integral role in educating state legislators. This led to rewriting North Dakota state century codes, differentiating hemp CBD from marijuana.

Renita created the international bestseller DVD "Game On" series for a billion-dollar network marketing company.

Renita is a sought-after public speaker with 2500+ presentations helping others take back control of their health, nutrition, and fitness.

Renita started a company called All Strong Moms — a program focused on education and empowerment to support moms in raising the next generation of leaders.

Her current health-related passion is to educate and empower others to apply cutting-edge, affordable phototherapy strategies.

This applied knowledge has changed millions of lives! It will change yours.

Ready to step into the light and start patching with phototherapy?

Order here:
www.lifewave.com/joyjoyjoy

Follow me here: www.facebook.com/renita.brannan

Connect with me via email at:
renewcoaching@yahoo.com

Kelly Brogan

WHEN AND HOW DID YOU FIRST DISCOVER THAT THE BODY HAS THE INNATE ABILITY TO HEAL ITSELF?

I was diagnosed after my first pregnancy with my first health condition that had the potential to become a chronic recidivistic, ongoing experience with the allopathic medical system—Hashimoto's thyroiditis. Because I had a lot of experience at that point treating women who had that diagnosis, I knew what conventional medicine had to offer me and I was not interested. I was simply uninterested in taking a prescription down to CVS every month for the rest of my life knowing that I would never really feel well again.

I decided at that moment, when I was presented the fork in the road of my journey, to travel into the unknown, and I sought a naturopath. I changed some significant lifestyle factors, including my diet, and I watched in black and white, on paper, my labs return to the normal range within one year. That made me a believer. I needed to walk a bridge of science from the conditioning and programming I had invested in my own medical training to a place of understanding that the body has the innate intelligence and wisdom to regulate itself and return to homeostasis. So I decided to devote my career for the rest of my life to honoring, healing, and exposing and curating the science that tells a different story about the body and the fact our symptoms are revealing to us an opportunity and an invitation to come into balance in ways we have not previously appreciated were even relevant.

WHY DO YOU THINK IT'S SO IMPORTANT FOR PEOPLE TO BE AWARE OF HOW THE BODY HEALS ITSELF?

I was one of the first three hundred psychiatrists to specialize in reproductive psychiatry, which was focused on prescribing psychotropic medication to pregnant and breastfeeding women. I became very aware of the importance of informed consent. In our medical training, of course, informed consent is a phrase we are familiarized with; however, it means to make a weighty decision examining all of the available evidence for the purported benefits, any risks, and the alternatives. It is the only way a patient can be properly empowered to navigate their health experience.

At this point I do not believe informed consent is available through the allopathic system, and maybe that is by design. Maybe we are in a moment where we are meant to self-source the information we need to make a decision in alignment with our highest expression, our personal development, and our psycho-spiritual maturation. But the informed consent model inspires me to make sure people have access to information about what is possible so they can feel magnetized toward their "yes." A lot of the time, when we are afraid we have symptoms and we are newly diagnosed, we have no energy. We reject what is happening. We say, "Not this. Give me the escape hatch. There has to be a way out." We fail to move into the next chapter of our life because we are attracted by this prospect of an escape and the possibility of what an answer to this question of illness might yield.

I have dedicated a lot of my resources to making sure people are aware of what is possible, that radical healing is possible. "Here is the documented case. Here is the published case. Here is the randomized trial." If you know it is possible, then your yes can ignite within you. And if you do not know something is possible, then you do not have a choice in the matter.

WHAT ADVICE DO YOU HAVE FOR CREATING HEALTH AND VITALITY FROM THE INSIDE OUT?

I have studied what I now see as the individuation journey of self-actualization over many years, and I have organized the stages, which are rather archetypal, into a three-part model—Get Real, Get Well, Get Free.

The **Get Real** phase of the journey is the mindset shift. In my protocol "vital mind reset," the first two weeks of the forty-four-day protocol are dedicated to reverse brainwashing. We make sure you are saturated with an entirely different worldview that centers your experience in your own narrative and infuses it with meaning. You gain an understanding of the why. "Why is this happening to me?" You are no longer functioning from a victim perspective but from the sovereign perspective. "Here is my why. Here is why I am being called to the carpet in this way, in this moment in time, in my lineage," in all the contextual details that are relevant.

When you develop that curiosity, it becomes an antidote to fear. You see there are thousands of studies that can help you understand the ways in which radical healing is possible through natural and lifestyle medicine. You see there is a bait and switch around conventional medicine offerings, specifically pharmaceuticals. You will then be able to reframe your psyche, and the rest of what happens is predicated on your nervous system, which is now oriented toward regeneration instead of fight, flight, and freeze.

The **Get Well** phase is behavioral change. It is the masculine initiation within. It is your inner father showing up inside of you to say, "I've got this. I am going to take the wheel. I am going to drive this car." And you exercise your power of choice, your integrity of word, and your capacity for commitment and follow-through. That is why I believe there is a ritual necessary. I have a 30-Day Reset protocol. There are many, many rituals available. You show up, you confront what you have been avoiding by your own decision-making, and you recognize that your choices matter. What you eat for breakfast matters. What time you go to bed matters. Every single one of your choices matters. This is the beginning of the transfer of the locus of control in your life within yourself instead of without.

The **Get Free** is how you begin to explore all of the bondage you have set up for yourself because you thought that was the only way for you to stay safe — all of the relationships, work environments, secrets — all the ways you are living small and stuck in your victim story. The untangling of those knots becomes very possible on an emotional level and on a physical level because your nervous system now has the capacity to allow you to move emotions like shame through your system so you can begin to reclaim the parts of yourself you never even knew were in hiding. This is the experience of coming home to ourselves that I think describes the destiny we all feel is possible within us at all stages of our lives.

About the Author

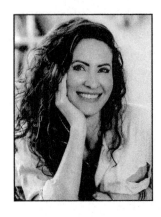

Kelly Brogan, M.D. is a holistic psychiatrist; author of the *New York Times* bestselling book, *A Mind of Your Own, Own Your Self;* the children's book, *A Time for Rain;* and co-editor of the landmark textbook *Integrative Therapies for Depression*. She is the founder of the online healing program Vital Mind Reset and the membership community, Vital Life Project. She completed her psychiatric training and fellowship at New York University Medical Center after graduating from Cornell University Medical College and has a Bachelor of Science from M.I.T. in Systems Neuroscience. She is specialized in a root-cause resolution approach to psychiatric syndromes and symptoms.

You can learn more about Dr. Kelly Brogan at www. kellybroganmd.com

Kim D'Eramo

WHEN AND HOW DID YOU FIRST DISCOVER THAT THE BODY HAS THE INNATE ABILITY TO HEAL ITSELF?

During medical school, I developed a strange illness no one could treat. I had severe joint pains, muscle spasms, shooting pains down my arms and legs, fatigue, and flu-like symptoms that persisted for months and months. I went to dozens of doctors and underwent all kinds of evaluations. I was put on several medications and remedies, including antidepressants, simply because no doctor could figure this out.

I had understood the *mind over matter* concept and that the body heals itself, so I tried harder and harder to change things to make this illness resolve. Nothing worked. Instead, I found that the harder I tried to heal, the more complicated my symptoms became.

Finally, I ended up in the office of one of Harvard University's best immunologists. He tested me for every allergen they had a test for, and I turned out to be "allergic" to almost all of them.

"Here's your answer! You have an autoimmune disease," I was told this, as if it were a sufficient answer. He said my condition would deteriorate, I would have to take medications for life and tightly control my living environment, and I would likely never run again.

I nearly turned into a puddle on the floor until I realized: *Wait a minute, is this really true for me?* I immediately felt a sense of strength and lightness. I thanked the doctor, exited the office, and decided to have a long listen to what my body really had to tell me.

That afternoon as I walked on the beach, I let go of all the fight and fear. I relaxed and gently asked my body to show me what it was trying to help me see. Rather than fighting the disease, fixing my problem, or trying to figure things out, I surrendered. I stopped asking: *What's wrong with me?* and started to ask: *What's right about this I'm not getting?*

I trusted and listened. I became a receiver instead of a doer. What happened next changed my life.

I suddenly became aware of all the years I'd been toiling away trying to excel and achieve, improve myself, and become a better person. I'd spent years working to overcome my circumstances and not let anything keep me down. Out of a deep fear of failure and an innate sense of personal inadequacy, I'd been living on the foundation of fight and battle. My body was simply showing me the reflection of that so I could see what this perspective was creating.

I realized my symptoms were not a punishment, as I'd come to see them, and not something to overcome or triumph beyond, but were a gentle message and invitation to release the faulty premise I was unsafe, unloved, and inadequate.

Wow! I thought. It was so clear, and part of me had been aware of this all along, but I had refused to really see it. In that moment, I entered a new relationship with my body. I finally surrendered the *fight* I had conjured up inside myself. I softened my body, let smooth full breaths flow in and out, and I was free.

Almost immediately my body healed fully from my symptoms. My labs returned to normal, and I became disease-free.

This forever changed the way I understood healing and gave me even more passion for my practice of medicine. I understood the scientific basis for how the mind and body are connected and how the body heals itself. I had integrated the experience of what it takes to create this. I had let into my own embodiment the inner connection of trust and surrender that allows Life Force to course through us more fully so the body can live disease-free.

This is an essential component to assisting others. It's not what we learn, but *who we are* that allows the healing to happen for us. It's not our credentials or degrees, but the consciousness we are in that allows us to *be the medicine.*

WHY DO YOU THINK IT'S SO IMPORTANT FOR PEOPLE TO BE AWARE OF HOW THE BODY HEALS ITSELF?

Since that day on the beach, I've seen my patients through a new lens. I created a medical practice based on the body's ability to heal itself and have focused on doing everything I can to assist that. I've witnessed my patients and clients heal from autoimmune diseases, Hashimoto's thyroiditis, multiple sclerosis (M.S.), cancer, severe pain syndromes like reflex sympathetic dystrophy (RSD), anxiety and depression, chronic fatigue syndrome, and many, many other conditions, some not even named in current medical understanding.

I've taught people all over the world the power of self-healing and how to unlock it. I've shown others how we are all connected to the Life Force, the Source energy that created us and creates us, and how to allow Source energy in more fully. I'm aware what we see as disease is only a reflection of what happens when we close down to the flow of Life Force, and that disease is not a thing to fight.

This ability to connect with Source has also greatly served my life, money, and relationships. I've witnessed for myself, and those I've worked with, profound and lasting healing in relationships and with money that had previously seemed impossible. Money showed up unexpectedly to meet dire needs, just as surrender and trust had been embraced. Children recovered from strange diseases, suicidality, or severe behavioral problems after healing had occurred within a parent. There are no conditions I've seen outside the realm of what can be healed and resolved when we connect with this power within.

I've fully dedicated my life to the practice of this medicine—conscious medicine—which incorporates the awareness healing happens from within, health and well-being are our natural state, and we are all connected.

WHAT ADVICE DO YOU HAVE FOR CREATING HEALTH AND VITALITY FROM THE INSIDE OUT?

Rather than the complexity of solutions that attempt to heal a disease or treat symptoms, the inner surrender to Source allows a sometimes instantaneous healing of any and every thing going awry in the body. The Source of Life that creates us already knows exactly what is needed and how to bring about the physiologic, electromagnetic changes to allow that. Instead of us doing the work, we *allow* the work to be done. Instead of trying harder and learning more, we can simply open to allow Life Force to come through more fully.

The space of Source does the rest. We do not need to earn it, deserve it, or even understand it; we just have to allow it, and it's ours.

We've been looking outside ourselves for the source, the medicine, the healer, and it just creates more problems to chase after. We won't find the real solutions out there. All of our hardships point us to this truth. When we awaken, we begin to see it is *the Life Force within ourselves* that we are seeking. When we connect with that, the I AM we truly are, all healing is possible. I'm grateful to have shared this work all over the world through my book *The MindBody Toolkit*, my weekly MindBody TV broadcast, my group courses and workshops, and my online home study courses. I'm blessed to have witnessed unthinkable healings every day! I've followed my own heart to allow the creation of my dream: to share this truth with others and change the face of medicine. If I can live this miracle, you can too! From my greatest pits of despair and doubt, I've again and again emerged, stronger and more sourced, centered and more whole. This is a process I live every day, and I continue to witness miracles of healing, of relationships, of money, and of creation.

I look forward to sharing this work with you for your own heart's desires to be manifest!

About the Author

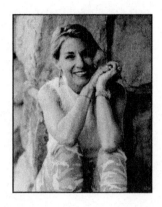

KIM D'ERAMO, D.O. is a physician, bestselling author of *The MindBody Toolkit*, and founder of DrKimD.com. She attended residency at Emory University and received her board certification in Emergency Medicine. Dr. D'Eramo has studied and practiced MindBody Medicine for decades after having experienced a severe anxiety disorder and later a severe autoimmune disease. She resolved both through self-healing after doctors told her she would be on medications for life. Kim now assists individuals and wellness practitioners all over the world to resolve illnesses and access the highest possibilities for vitality and abundance. She shares a weekly live international MindBody TV broadcast, and she can be found at DrKimD.com.

You can get her bestselling book *The MindBody Toolkit* at DrKimD.com/book and begin your own healing journey with her powerful course *The Instant Elevation* at DrKimD.com/iep to raise your personal frequency and heal disease.

Stephanie Dobranski

WHEN AND HOW DID YOU FIRST DISCOVER THAT THE BODY HAS THE INNATE ABILITY TO HEAL ITSELF?

In 2004, I began having dreams that inspired me to spend a tremendous amount of time in nature. My dreams were images of birds, streams, and scenes in nature. Upon waking, I would look out the window to see hawks or owls scouring in the branches. On one occasion, a hawk landed on a nearby branch and looked at me, neither of us flinching. It felt as if he were looking directly into my eyes. I received images of places to go in nature; then I would go to those locations and find feathers, and I would sit with them. It would be the feather of the bird which came to the window that morning.

I took walks along the nearby Potomac River and found Native American artifacts along the path. One day, my bones felt as if they were heating up and my body began to vibrate. This compelled me to quicken my pace through the woods. My eyes filled with tears, and I fell down at the base of a tree, crying uncontrollably.

There I released all my old emotional trauma. My body responded with a wisdom flowing within me. I discovered my body had the ability to heal itself by being in silence and within nature, and that is a very powerful tool.

Nature was beginning to speak to me. The trees and flowers would say something like a lion or like a flower would say something. I would go home and look up the message, and it would be an herb and I would start taking it.

My walks continued. I would seek out a tree to sit under for a while, and the trauma would be completely cleared out of me. Spending time in nature transformed my life and my body because I was releasing emotions. The tree became the mother I never had. The warm earth hugged me. I was encircled in the Mother's healing love.

The vibrational feelings helped me feel clear, with no spinning thoughts in my head. I knew there was an intelligence to the earth and within my physical body because of the way it would shake or move or guide me to a certain tree or location. That is how nature started communicating and healing me, and how I started understanding the divine design within the intelligence of the body. Yes, from dreams, to following the guidance, to the birds—some kind of intelligence made the birds come to me. I would see an image and know where to go because I knew the land. This went on for a very long time.

WHY DO YOU THINK IT'S SO IMPORTANT FOR PEOPLE TO BE AWARE OF HOW THE BODY HEALS ITSELF?

When people realize they are divine design and intelligence, they take their power back. They take their freedom back. They take their life back. They take their finances back into their control. They take back their ability to create within this world. When people realize it is all within them — a beautiful design and intelligence — they can reclaim their power, life force, and ability to create. Healing is just the beginning. After healing, there is a whole world for them to explore.

Once that light switch comes on, a door opens up to magic. Realize your body has the ability to heal itself and swim in the field of intelligence. The best way to tap into this is through nature, which will cause everything to shift very quickly. The body is activated. Your mind is activated, allowing healing and transformation to take place as soon as you become aware it is even possible. That is why people should go in nature.

This process put the magic back in my life. It rekindled the fire and took me away from desperation and fear. I no longer wanted to give up. I didn't fall into the pain — physical or emotional.

WHAT ADVICE DO YOU HAVE FOR CREATING HEALTH AND VITALITY FROM THE INSIDE OUT?

First, acknowledge your body's divine design and intelligence. Second, trust in that and be open to receiving the internal guidance directing you toward exploring more deeply. Work with people who support you in finding the modalities calling to you through ancient healing arts, herbs, or Qi Gong frequency tools. Modalities are advertised within the realm of the 3D, but they are really ancient wisdom from the forest, trees, and streams — nature.

Spend time in nature. Be open to things you have never tried before. Be open to feeling your way into modalities that seem off the wall. You have to acknowledge you automatically walk the same way, you automatically write the same way, and you automatically drive or wipe your nose after you sneeze the same way. All these automatic forces that flow through you are just the first step to understanding the intelligence of the body. Your body automatically does these things. When you start opening to realms and fields and energies, just the thought of a tuning fork, a singing bowl, neuro feedback, herbs, talking to a tree — just opening to those thoughts will cause the body to resonate into a field of knowledge. The body organically wants to function optimally. The body will be optimized all the time if it is allowed.

We are divinely intelligent. Our body wants to be an Olympic athlete. The intelligence we are wants to automatically optimize itself. When we engage, just for a brief moment, in smoke gazing, fire gazing, bark gazing, watching the river flow — the body will instantly click into optimization. The more and more you allow the body to optimize itself, the more you realize your divine design.

Acknowledge your body's divine design and intelligence, spend time in nature, and work with people who support you in finding the energies that enhance your divine design. Investigate herbs, ancient healing arts like Qi Gong, martial arts, and toning. Research frequency tools like Neuro Biofeedback. By recognizing and acknowledging the body has the ability to heal itself by divine design intelligence, you will reclaim your power, life force, freedom, and money.

About the Author

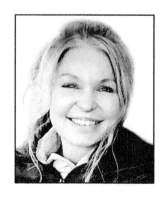

For the last twenty years, Stephanie has traveled an extraordinary path to discovery of the many dimensions available to all in every breath, every thought, and every choice. Using ancient and modern metaphysical tools and technology, Stephanie's primary teacher has been her deep connection and communication with the wisdom and healing powers of Mother Earth and the animal kingdom. She is cultivated in the application of transformational tools such as non-linear neurofeedback, Chi Gong, herbs, sound frequencies, the Akashic records, nature bathing, and the healing power of animals. These modalities brought her to the determination of holographic fields as malleable, permeable intelligence in which we live. This leads to an evolving understanding that humanity accesses and constantly communicates with other fields of intelligence and conscious beings.

Get in touch with Stephanie's services, tools, and modalities at http://www.33minutestozen.com.

Susan Green

WHEN AND HOW DID YOU FIRST DISCOVER THAT THE BODY HAS THE INNATE ABILITY TO HEAL ITSELF?

I have lived with a lifetime of pain since I was very, very young. When I hit my thirties and went through some traumatic stages, I came down with a lot of chronic fatigue to the point it was very debilitating on every level of life. I could not think or function — physically, metaphysically, energetically, emotionally, or mentally. In my early forties, I woke up one day and decided I was not going to live like that anymore. I do not even know how that decision came forth.

I had been reading about past lives, which always fascinated me, and I went down to a local crystal shop and asked if there was anyone who could do a past life regression and met an energy healer. She started doing energy sessions on me, and my response was phenomenal. Every time I had a session, I would be completely wiped out, but my body releasing was awakening me. At the same time, I created a path of recognizing how food, lifestyle, grounding, meditation, and reconnecting with the insight of who I am was healing me. I accelerated very quickly from absolute fog and disability into being able to live and function on a whole new level. It was absolutely amazing, after a lifetime of trying to find answers, this was so easy—just by understanding the influences of energy and reconnecting with the heart space, with self, and grounding with the life we are living.

I quickly accelerated to understanding it was my purpose to bring this experience to other people because the response was so phenomenal and so powerful and so rapid. This very quickly developed into my own business using quantum healing, seeing the threads of life to transcend past, present, and future. It still amazes me to be able to say I am healing others after having lived with my own disability for so long. It is a living miracle the body can heal itself. When you understand the process, you can literally rewire all you are to become what you want to be when you do the right thing for your body by giving it all it needs.

WHY DO YOU THINK IT'S SO IMPORTANT FOR PEOPLE TO BE AWARE OF HOW THE BODY HEALS ITSELF?

What I believe and what I have experienced in my own journey is how the correlation of past influences, past lives, and emotional blocks were making me ill in this life. I have learned how to resolve them. So it was very much those threads of reality of the past healing and the ripple being created, which offset the blueprint I was living by and healed this life.

When people understand their history, as in karmic history, it empowers their momentum communicated through the collective being lived now and opens the mind to their potential. It opens them to a sense of purpose and passion. If you can heal from a disability into wellness of mind, body, and soul, then you suddenly find this correlates into a purpose, passion, and a desire to live and create the same for others, and it is communicated effortlessly. Suddenly life is not just a drag, so difficult, and a daily grind. It has a purpose and a passion that give you a desire to create. When you come from disability into wellness, you wake up every day saying to yourself, "This is amazing! If only more people could realize how amazing this gift of life is."

It is all about understanding, "Ah, now I know why that relationship is not working." Or "Now I know why I feel this way because that has been my karmic pattern." When you reconcile a trauma and heal energy and emotion from an organ, body system, or energy pathway, all of a sudden everything else starts feeling so much better. The transition and transformation are phenomenal on every level. When you understand how the body heals itself, you understand appreciation, gratitude, and self-love. Those things are pivotal in everything else you do and help you feel worthy and accepted. To be aware of how the body can heal itself is the most phenomenal thing in all aspects of bringing back unity.

WHAT ADVICE DO YOU HAVE FOR CREATING HEALTH AND VITALITY FROM THE INSIDE OUT?

This is about living and activating life through the heart and not just thinking with the head. Obviously, you have to live with a certain amount of conscious choice and understanding that the radiating ego mind and emotional self, which radiate in the head, really cloud judgment. When you activate your heart and think with your heart instead of your head, you open your consciousness in appreciation and gratitude of self, others, and the planet we are living on, and that keeps rippling out.

You become committed to the vision of good health without excuses. All of a sudden you are not living in justification. The greatest advice I can give is to not make excuses as to why you cannot do it. Make the decision and commit to yourself because you are important. You are worth the effort. You are so valuable. Your light will start to shine, and you will go from a dim state of being unwell to gaining momentum and getting brighter and brighter and brighter. Soon the fog is no longer there, the mental looping is no longer happening, and you'll see the details. You'll see the trees instead of just the forest. You'll see the tiniest bugs having a little party time on flowers because it is so beautiful. You'll understand how joyous life really can be.

Appreciation and gratitude help you notice the details and live in the vision of good health without excuses. It is committing to yourself when you say, "I am worth it. I am enough. I believe I can do this." Make the tough choices to actually do it. Commit to that. Be aware of living in a higher perspective so you do not get caught up in the messiness. Let go of what does not serve you anymore so you can truly step forward. You will see not everything is a personal attack and you do not need to be radiating in negative energy. Let it go and understand what is important and what is not important in a higher perspective. See all the influences so you can make positive decisions, without getting into negative turmoil. Remember the heart space. Live through the heart, not the head.

About the Author

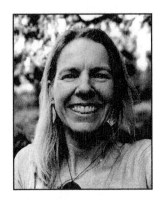

Susan Green – Visionary Force and Inspiration Behind Airmeith

As a psychic and medical medium, Susan possesses the ability to access the webs of reality that intricately link lifetimes. Seamlessly weaving the threads of the past, present, and future, Susan reveals the convergence in the present that shapes your existence. She discerns the resistance and densities that shifted you from your divine source blueprint. She explains how these deviations disrupt the optimal communication of your light code (DNA), in turn affecting your physical health, mental clarity, emotional equilibrium, and intuitive insight.

Susan employs divine frequencies to initiate transformative corrections within the matrix of existence. This involves updating the resonance, shape, and structure of your life force like a potent quantum healing cocktail harmoniously blended to achieve remarkable results, shared by many who have experienced profound change, as showcased on her website.

One-on-one healing sessions and mentoring services involve the use of pendulums, animal oracles, and dowsing charts. These and other tools serve as beacons of empowerment on your soul journey, guiding you toward a reality that previously felt beyond your wildest dreams.

Susan is your catalyst for transformation, beckoning you to boldly step into the boundless potential of your own existence.

"I truly want to help all people experience the miracles I have. I want to help them live in the freedom that I do. I have this beautiful ability, which I never knew about. I want to bring that light and awaken that light within other people. If you would like to work with me, please reach out through my contact information below."

https://www.healwithairmeith.com/

https://linktr.ee/healwithairmeith

Michele T. Griffith

WHEN AND HOW DID YOU FIRST DISCOVER THAT THE BODY HAS THE INNATE ABILITY TO HEAL ITSELF?

I received a form of myofascial bodywork called Body Memory Recall (BMR) from Jonathan A. Tripodi in 2021. I had a lengthy list of physical and emotional complaints on my intake, and within three days I noticed changes I had wanted for years. I was sleeping through the night, had clear thoughts, peace, and acceptance about events from my past, and a way to work with my thoughts, emotions, and sensations to release stress. The experience helped me integrate a new understanding of myself as a self-resourced person.

As a self-resourced person, I have tools and knowledge to care for my body, mind, and soul. I also have curiosity and assertiveness skills to ask for additional skills when I realize it is time to learn more. Sometimes *assertiveness skills* lead me to recognize my limits, set boundaries that work for me, and discern next steps forward in personal and work realms.

WHY DO YOU THINK IT'S SO IMPORTANT FOR PEOPLE TO BE AWARE OF HOW THE BODY HEALS ITSELF?

Awareness of how the body works allows the power and freedom to be rightfully within the person's facilitation. I had relied upon physicians, hospitals, therapists, mentors, gurus, and even relationships for guidance and answers to my body's mysteries. When I finally accepted that I possess my own blueprint for health, I had a revelation of confidence and awe. My blueprint includes listening deeply to what is happening to my body; trusting my own inner inclinations; using intentional breath, stretches, and mindfulness to work with sensations; and other forms of expression such as journaling, artwork, body movement, and meditation.

This self-reliance experience revolutionized my personal history and transformed how I work with clients. I trust their inner realms and what their symptoms are speaking to them. In my past, I sometimes wanted to "cure" unwanted symptoms and make them disappear. In 2021, I found courage to be in conversation with whatever arises in me and now this is exactly the treatment that results in positive outcomes for others.

When clients create inner space to face their own symptoms, they often spontaneously arrive at insights and conclusions that make sense to them, and soon they are mastering their intuitive knowledge of the next steps for their healing. It is the reward of a lifetime to observe someone end treatment in a state of empowerment, enthusiasm, and inspiration.

WHAT ADVICE DO YOU HAVE FOR CREATING HEALTH AND VITALITY FROM THE INSIDE OUT?

Never give up the dream of creating vital health. As I look back at my own history, I see glimpses of what I learned in 2021 from BMR to create the space of listening, trust, and love for myself. I was aware of my inner space at times during childhood, and I had a profound experience in a therapist's office during a guided visualization at age twenty-one. However, I did not trust myself. I felt unrest, startled, and unsure if these experiences were "normal." In my thirties and forties, I learned a formal meditation practice and skills for art therapy and counseling as a social worker. I found bodywork and continued subconscious mind and energy dynamics exploration in my fifties to finally make peace with my inner space.

This relationship with my inner realm has been the most rewarding experience for my health and well-being. I use my inner awareness to scan my body with a gentle attitude and curiosity — especially from the top of my head to my navel, where I regularly experience the majority of my thoughts and feelings. I commit to myself with loving kindness affirmations such as, "This inner space is the friendliest place on Earth for me." I release tension or stress at the end of every day with body movement, tears, writing, or verbalizing with close friends. I continue to discern appropriate actions with my precious life that support myself and others in my community. I celebrate reasons to smile and laugh and count the wins of the day. Today, I am in the practice of living into my dream life.

About the Author

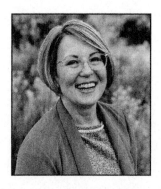

Michele T. Griffith, MFA, MS, MSW is in the practice of living her dream life. She is an author and speaker and collaborator. In her private practice, Art in Motion (AIM) for Wellness, she creates successful outcomes for clients facing mood, trauma, or relationship distress. She is an author and speaker and collaborator. She travels with her brother, Bill Griffith, creator of the *Cope, Hope, or Dope* podcast, and Cinda Robison, author and co-creator of wellness workshops for schools and organizations. Michele, Bill, and Cinda create customized wellness workshops based on the needs of their audience, which include how to utilize intentional breath for wellness, unique mindfulness and meditation strategies, mind-body connection education, emotional regulation, and stress management.

Michele developed her eclectic approach by spending time in academia learning Rhetoric, Art Therapy, and Social Work at the master's level from 2001–2011 and received her clinical certification in social work in 2019. In counseling, the communication training, the creativity, and the mental health interventions connected full circle. Mental health combined with healing and transformation philosophies, gave way to new whole-body approaches: body, mind, and soul. Michele spent a year learning Body Memory Recall, created by Jonathan A. Tripodi, a healing modality for releasing trauma from body tissues. Michele is currently taking a deeper dive into working with sensitive soul modalities created by Dr. Karen Kan, Academy of Light Medicine and energetic modalities created by Marcus Bird and the Centre for Quantum Healing. When Michele is not working, she creates artwork, writes; and enjoys hiking, water sports, and travel.

What is the barrier you have identified to your vital health and well-being? Can you name it fully here?

Barrier:

Is it a physical or emotional ailment? Can you imagine trusting there is a path toward healing it fully? Can you imagine what your life would be like if you busted through these identified barriers? Write down five actions you would like to take with your renewed precious life, as if they are happening now, enabling you to step into your dream life. Now you are filled with vital health and well-being:

1.

2.

3.

4.

5.

Share your five actions with me at my Facebook or email address:

Art In Motion (AIM) Facebook:

https://www.facebook.com/ artinmotionaimforwellness

Email: ArtInMotionAIMforWellness@gmail.com

I offer a free thirty-minute consultation about your list of preferred living. In that consultation, you will learn next steps for working with yourself and receive at least one resource to explore for more information. Send me an email or Facebook message with BOOK OFFER in the heading, and I will respond within twenty-four hours to arrange a consultation at a convenient day and time for you.

I am working with my brother, Bill, and a friend and colleague, Cinda, to create the Wellness Workshop now touring. To inquire about custom Wellness Workshops for your organization with Bill K. Griffith, Michele Griffith, and Cinda Robison, visit:

Bill K. Griffith:
https://billkgriffith.com/
https://www.facebook.com/bill.griffith.12

Cinda K. Robison:
https://www.empath.expert/
coaching2heal@gmail.com

Michele T Griffith:
Email: ArtInMotionAIMforWellness@gmail.com

I'd love to have a conversation about your dream life!

Holly Hallowell

WHEN AND HOW DID YOU FIRST DISCOVER THAT THE BODY HAS THE INNATE ABILITY TO HEAL ITSELF?

When I think back to when I first discovered the body's incredible capacity to heal itself, I'm brought back to 2014 — a painful period of loss in my life that ultimately led to profound growth. I had just lost my job and was struggling to patch together an income while caring for my young daughter. The layers of stress weighed heavy. I developed high blood pressure and thyroid issues, and I gained weight. I was handed prescription after prescription, as traditional medicine seemed focused on temporarily masking symptoms rather than nurturing the root causes for true healing.

I knew there had to be a better way. I yearned to understand my body more deeply. That inner knowing led me to explore holistic modalities like acupuncture, herbs, and breathwork. As I learned concepts like energy flow and reconnecting to restore balance, things began to shift. My symptoms lessened; my outlook lifted. With each small healing, it felt like my body was remembering its innate wisdom.

The more I studied, the more a singular truth emerged: At our core, we are all connected energy and information. When we realign to the memory of that unity held within every cell, miraculous healing unfolds. Resonating with the Divine energy that flows through all, I witnessed my body repair itself on the most profound levels. Stress melted away, blood pressure normalized, and the thyroid balanced. I gently weaned myself off each medication after a few months. When I went back for medical testing, every marker glowed with vitality.

In that moment, the doctor's puzzlement over my progress crystallized something for me — true healing arises from within. When we tune inward and reconnect with our wholeness, we tap into the body's spectacular symphony of self-regeneration. I emerged transformed by this awakening, devoted to supporting others in harmonizing with their own healing potential. Our bodies hold far more wisdom than we can imagine — we need only listen.

WHY DO YOU THINK IT'S SO IMPORTANT FOR PEOPLE TO BE AWARE OF HOW THE BODY HEALS ITSELF?

It's vital for us to recognize the body's inherent wisdom — its spectacular capacity to heal itself when given the chance. For too long, we have relinquished our personal power, allowing the medical machine to dictate symptoms and treatments without tuning into root causes. Our bodies hold far more genius than the system gives credit.

When we take time to peel back the layers and sit with our whole, imperfect selves, we reconnect to an inner healer waiting to be heard. It's important to continually remind ourselves that well-being isn't found in sterilized labs; it's been inside us all along, coded into each brilliant cell. Pharmaceuticals can only manipulate what the body already knows at its core.

Of course, sometimes expert care is essential. But what if we made it standard practice to partner with professionals instead of handing away the reins? Help them understand us as complex humans with endless potential for self-repair. Guide them in strategically supporting our innate healing response rather than forcing change based solely on textbooks and unbalanced incentives.

Neuroplasticity is scientifically proven; our brains can form new neural connections throughout life. That means we have the incredible capacity to shift out of limiting patterns into mental spaces that serve our highest purpose. When stress, trauma, or toxic messaging locks our nervous system into fear-based circuits, we can consciously rewire new courageous pathways instead. By leaning into our discomfort with curiosity and self-compassion, we practice emotional agility to move through shame and vulnerability. As we uncover and write bold new stories of self-worth and agency, we can transform old tales of "never enough." This reclamation of authority over our inner world awakens the mind's spectacular power to manifest well-being aligned with our whole, authentic selves.

My hope is that through radical self-awareness and community, we will unlock access to the healer within each of us. But first, we must nurture the humility to admit when we feel lost and dare to wonder who we might become by trusting in our body's infinite wisdom once more.

WHAT ADVICE DO YOU HAVE FOR CREATING HEALTH AND VITALITY FROM THE INSIDE OUT?

True health blossoms from within. You already have everything you need within you. Society will try to convince you healing comes from the latest gadget or pill, but your vitality has been intricately coded into every cell, patiently waiting to be awakened.

So how do we tap into that power? It starts by nurturing your connection to the Divine, however you may define it. Make sacred space for stillness; bathe your senses in nature; meditate to live fully in the only time we have, which is this moment. As you quiet external noise, soften into your body's innate wisdom.

When we rush around the clock without pause, pushing ourselves past exhaustion, it cracks our gentle foundation. Our nervous systems strain under chronic stress, unable to reset. Make it a priority to rest, restore, and ground yourself regularly. Sleep enough to infuse your days with spark and clarity. Move your body in ways that ignite passion, not punishment. Fuel yourself with wholesome, delicious food while also tuning into more subtle nutritional needs unique to your makeup. Drink more water; its cleansing life force heals at a cellular level.

It is just as important to carefully curate your emotional ecosystems as it is to make healthy lifestyle choices. Limit time around those who energize your inner critic. Instead, nurture community that celebrates your voice and spirit. Protect your energy by rejecting messages that weaponize shame or scarcity; those profound lies thrive when we feel unworthy. Have the courage to walk away from environments misaligned with your soul. It is sacred self-care.

When we make space to connect to our authentic essence, creativity flows freely once more. And here is the secret: Creativity is integral medicine lighting up every cell. Make creativity a vital part of your self-care routine, whether through art, writing, dance, or anything that sparks cathartic joy. Follow those effervescent callings. Fully living your purpose exponentially nourishes health, giving you a reason to live. When you have purpose, you have the longevity to get there.

We can also consciously harness the power of vibration to shift our health. For example, when we code water with frequencies attuned to particular goals — whether it's improved immunity, energy, detoxification, or other aims — we infuse every sip with a specific vibrational essence. As that water integrates throughout our tissues, it raises our cellular vibration to resonate with more vibrant states in remarkably tangible ways. Much like a tuning fork setting off ripples of its matching tone, we can use water's receptive nature as a tool to amplify targeted energetic patterns already flowing through us. This instantly elevates baseline wellness. Through intentionally leveraging vibration, we direct our transformational capability and sync up with pure prana and our full potential.

Finally, in those moments we lose our way, respond with loving kindness. Start by receiving your whole self exactly as you are now. Perfection is not required. Healing happens through practicing courage and compassion moment by moment. When you stumble on this journey of radical self-love, do not spiral into shame. Instead, nurture acceptance and patience within your perfectly imperfect humanity. Gently realign to your resilience, remembering you have everything within to find your way. You will rise again and again, living wholeheartedly through the ebbs and flows. Embracing all of who you are with grace is what ultimately reclaims your power. When self-love sinks into your bones, you walk this world unshakeable, aglow with inner vitality. You tap into the infinite fountain of health flowing through you, awakened to your sovereignty once more.

About the Author

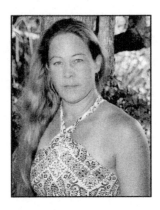

Holly Hallowell (Anahata)

In 2015, a divine download transformed my life, bridging the Law of Attraction with energy medicine through the channeling of the Anahata Codes. Over the past decade, I've witnessed these transformative Codes help countless individuals transcend limitations, heal deeply, and discover their true life purpose.

As founder of the Alchemical Academy, I've cultivated an online haven where our community of Manifesting Luminaries learns, grows, and manifests magic together, supported by expert mentors offering invaluable insights through transformational courses.

Drawing from past-life memories as a Waterbender in ancient Lumeria, I've unearthed the lost wisdom of water science—knowledge that empowers us to tap into water's vibrational magic and use it as a wand to manifest desires.

My mission is to guide each soul to unparalleled joy as author of their life. Let's weave timelines where passion intertwines seamlessly with purpose for your fulfillment and planetary contribution.

My journey has also inspired me to author four bestselling books, with four more underway. Check out my author profile on Amazon to explore my body of literary work.

Harness inner alchemy by joining the Alchemical Academy, full of free resources on activating well-being through nature's resonance: www.Alchemical.Academy.

Subscribe to our YouTube channel to align with your sovereign power and manifest dreams of health, wealth, purpose, and passion: @alchemical.academy.

https://www.youtube.com/channel/UCEjei5NyS3wi1FGSSEfdG3g

Sophia Harvey

WHEN AND HOW DID YOU FIRST DISCOVER THAT THE BODY HAS THE INNATE ABILITY TO HEAL ITSELF?

I was twenty-three years old and struggling with my physical health—polycystic ovarian syndrome, fibromyalgia, and irritable bowel syndrome, to name but a few challenges. It felt debilitating. Amongst my community, Western Medicine was considered the solution to all ailments. Accordingly, I sought the advice of various medical specialists. The outcome was diagnoses, drugs, and lifelong management plans.

Being a curious human, I decided to investigate alternatives. I wanted to find solutions that meant illness maintenance was a thing of the past. In my research, I discovered naturopathy, Traditional Chinese Medicine, and energetic healing modalities. Experimenting with these produced incredible results, with many symptoms disappearing.

A couple of years later in my professional Neuro-Linguistic Programming (NLP), Somatic Psychotherapy and Process-Oriented Psychology (POP) trainings, I discovered a key piece of the puzzle that felt critical. I discovered our emotions and thoughts deeply influence our bodily health. I had learned the basics regarding how the body is impacted through stress responses in my university psychology studies. Understanding, however, that stuck emotions and limiting thought patterns can be causally linked to presenting physical body issues was novel, exciting information. It was fascinating to learn firsthand, through my NLP and POP session practice, that the physical symptoms can therefore provide the entry point to discover and transform previously hidden psychological and emotional patterns holding us back from thriving.

A key example from my direct experience came through my attention to my polycystic ovaries (which were still symptomatic). I used my physical symptoms as the doorway to discover deeper, non-logical yet emotively true, limiting patterns stored within my ovaries, including "it's not safe to be a woman" and "you will be harmed if you speak your truth as a woman." I diligently engaged in practices to clear these patterns, acknowledging their origins were old, possibly beyond this lifetime. We only need to look at epigenetics to understand that we can inherit traumas, and thus limiting beliefs, ancestrally. After completing the processes, I felt lighter and there was no longer an emotive response in my body to those limiting pattern statements. A month later, an ultrasound revealed that my ovaries were clear of cysts and highly functional. They still are.

WHY DO YOU THINK IT'S SO IMPORTANT FOR PEOPLE TO BE AWARE OF HOW THE BODY HEALS ITSELF?

Imagine a world where you hold the key to your well-being, a place where the power to heal resides not just in external forces but within you, waiting to be awakened. This isn't a fantasy; it's the essence of understanding how your body heals itself.

For so long, many of us have relinquished control over our health, outsourcing to others' definitions of what it means to be healthy or successful. This shift away from self-trust has led to an increasingly disempowered population, where decisions are often made from a place of fear or based on what others think is best. When we make decisions from fear or societal pressures, the wisdom of our intuition, or our inner authority, is forgotten.

Imagine a reality where we understand that nobody knows our bodies and our needs better than we do. Each person's life journey is unique. There is no single formula that is a good fit for all. One person cannot say what's best for another. Only the individual knows this, as only that individual resides within their own body-mind. As humans, we learn and develop from our individual experiences, and sometimes the challenges provide us with incredible growth. Acknowledging our body's capacity for self-healing empowers us to tune into our inner voice, guiding us toward choices that truly serve our well-being. Whether it involves conventional medicine, natural remedies, energetic healing, psychological work, or a combination of these approaches, the guiding principle is following what genuinely aligns with our distinct path.

Trusting our intuitive knowing leads us into self-mastery, where we take responsibility for our lives, making discerning choices that facilitate our growth, expand our conscious awareness, and actualize our purpose. This journey of self-development builds a deep connection within and extends beyond us. It encourages us to delve into our inner world, shedding light on areas once enshrouded in darkness and fostering a profound understanding of our true essence. This path leads to a reconnection with ourselves, and also with the larger world, as we realize our symbiotic relationship with all that exists, underscoring our vital place within the natural order.

Our collective disconnection has manifested in numerous global challenges that have not only impacted our individual health, but also the well-being of our planet. By fostering this deeper symbiotic connectivity within us and between everything that breathes, we naturally embrace a position of responsibility and optimism, not just for our own health, but also for relational and environmental harmony.

Appreciating our symptoms as messages, as gentle nudges from our bodies seeking attention and care, allows us to shift from fighting disease to embracing a path of healing and understanding. Curiosity and loving acceptance of our body signals can occur, instead of us rejecting or suppressing them. Our symptoms of pain and discomfort can be seen as ways of supporting us to tune into and transform limiting patterns and outdated beliefs still stored within us. This inquiry process goes far beyond just treating symptoms, instead guiding us to their root cause, paving the way for authentic healing of body, mind, and spirit.

WHAT ADVICE DO YOU HAVE FOR CREATING HEALTH AND VITALITY FROM THE INSIDE OUT?

Expanding skills in self-awareness and presence is paramount. This will assist in noticing and understanding what is arising internally: emotionally, physically, and psychologically. Meditation can really support this development. Practices focusing on recognizing body signals will also be important. These may include body mapping and body sensation awareness exercises. Once the body signals have been pinpointed, the messages they are trying to communicate will need to be understood. It may be enough to tune into the body symptom and ask the question: "What are you trying to share with me?" However, a deeper process guided by a skilled professional may be required. Cultivation of intuitive listening is a key component of self-awareness development. A simple practice to support this is a daily nourishment task, asking the question: "What will nourish me today?" It is important to allow the response to arise through the body-mind and then commit to doing it, noticing how you feel when you listen to and act in accordance with this inner voice.

The body-mind needs to be treated as something sacred that requires nurturing to thrive. Listening to your answers to the following questions will support this self-care.

- What foods nourish your body?

- What liquids fuel it?

- What movement supports it?

- What thoughts love it?

- What attitudes respect it?

- What actions cherish it?

- What connections with others, with nature, and spirituality energize it?

- Do you need natural herbs or supplements to support it?

- Is your energetic field clear?

- If not, how can you get support with this?

- Are you grounded?

- If not, what can you do to change this?

- Are you taking time to play? Never underestimate the power of play to support health and healing.

It is essential to process what is arising emotionally and mentally. Bypassing emotions and undesired thoughts suppresses them and moves them into the subconscious system. These emotions and thoughts instead require kindhearted consideration, acceptance, and understanding before they can be released from the body-mind system. This inner work cannot be fast-tracked or avoided. Attending to these emergent patterns also means having honest conversations about your needs and challenges in relationships. If such communication is evaded, the issues will likely resurface in other ways, through emotional outbursts, avoidant behavior, or physical body symptoms. Outsourcing to holistic practitioners can again support this journey. We all have blind spots, so the trusted support of a skilled professional can assist in identification of the root issues whilst allowing us to surrender more deeply into the processes and practices designed to assist our healing.

Understanding the power of love to promote healing is imperative. I had an incredible experience of this when I was in a Cuban Intensive Care Unit, following a near-death vehicular accident. I will always remember the eleven medical practitioners looking at me with so much love in their eyes throughout my hospitalization. Their loving energy was palpable. I could feel it in my body. It instilled me with hope and gave me the strength to rise beyond the pain and tenderly focus my attention on healing. When I arrived in the USA, after two days in the Cuban ICU, the American medics were astounded at how much my body had already healed. I always credit a huge part of my healing to that love and care from the Cuban medical staff, in addition to the power of my own mind and my ability to access that loving vibration from within me.

When engaging in restorative well-being work, it is important to remain hopeful, even when it seems there is little to no change or improvement. Trusting the process of your health journey is crucial. I have only recently emerged from a significant chronic illness that began after a barrage of emotionally exhausting life challenges. It took me just over two years of working physically, psychologically, and energetically, identifying and clearing deeply buried patterns that I had been oblivious to. There were times that I wanted to give up, but I reminded myself of all the other times

I had healed. I kept bringing myself back to trust and reached out for support when I needed it.

We must remember when we heal and move through one layer, there are others within us that can emerge on different planes of our existence: physically, psychologically, emotionally, or energetically. When considering the depths of our souls and our interconnectedness as beings, it makes sense that healing and associated growth is a lifetime journey. The more we trust the process, the easier it becomes. The deeper we dive in, the more we metamorphose our lives into coherence and fulfilment.

About the Author

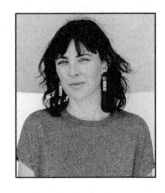

Sophia Harvey is a Holistic Psychologist and Leadership and Well-Being Specialist who is passionate about supporting people to live purposeful, aligned lives. With a background in psychology, criminal law, human rights, community development, and research, Sophia has a wealth of cross-cultural, international, and multidisciplinary experience that supports her to understand the depth and breadth of human experiences. She holds a Master's in Psychology, Honour's in Law, as well as numerous diplomas and certifications in coaching, psychotherapy, embodied movement, and energetic healing modalities. Sophia has published research papers and been a guest speaker at various conferences and training institutes regarding her psychology work. She is the co-author of an internationally best-selling book and has developed the Zebra Crossing Project™. It incorporates a number of courses and coaching pathways designed to support the "zebras" of the world—leaders and heart-centered humans wanting to create impactful change—to safely cross from the ordinary to the extraordinary in their life work. It is a deep journey cultivating authentic and intuitive living, to harness an empowered and ecologically purposeful life. Focusing on emotional, physical, mental and spiritual health to resolve root-cause issues, is crucial to this journey. In her spare time, she loves adventuring with her beloved cheeky pooch, dancing, and immersing herself in nature.

Courses: Live and Lead Series. Through embodied practice, you will learn to listen to your body signals, transform deep-rooted limiting patterns impacting optimal functioning and relating, whilst maximizing intuitive listening to support quintessential decision-making and purposeful, healthful living and leading.

Free resources: The Power of Presence Guide and The Intuition Archetype Quiz.

All accessible here: sophiaharvey.com

Bethany Miller, RN

WHEN AND HOW DID YOU FIRST DISCOVER THAT THE BODY HAS THE INNATE ABILITY TO HEAL ITSELF?

It has been referred to by various terms such as vitalism, natural healing, holistic health, and more. Nevertheless, we opt to label it *Innate Health*, as it encapsulates the inherent capability of your body to heal and safeguard itself. Consider this: from birth, our cells possess the innate knowledge of multiplication, and our bodies inherently understand the process of growth.

The Inspirational Journey of Holistic Healing and Unlocking the Power Within: In the intricate tapestry of our existence, a remarkable phenomenon unfolds — the body's innate ability to heal itself from the inside out, encompassing the realms of mind, body, and spirit. My journey of holistic healing is not merely a physical convalescence, but a transformative experience that taps into the profound depths of our being. As a registered nurse, I've consistently marveled at the paradox where some individuals, despite having promising prognoses, grapple with chronic illnesses and weakened immune systems. Conversely, there are numerous accounts of people facing stage 4 cancer or other severe ailments, yet they manage to heal and recover against formidable odds. My nursing journey has catapulted me into an empowering tale centered around the body's inherent ability to self-heal. It involves delving into the intricate interplay of the mind, body, and spirit, forming a harmonious symphony that contributes to overall well-being.

1. The Resilience of the Physical Body: At the heart of the body's healing prowess lies the extraordinary dance of cellular renewal. Each moment, trillions of cells collaborate in a symphony of growth, repair, and regeneration. This constant renewal ensures that the body sheds the old and embraces the new, a testament to its commitment to vitality and restoration. When everything is as it should be, the immune system, a stalwart guardian, stands ready to defend against external invaders. Its ceaseless vigilance and adaptability showcase the body's capacity to overcome challenges. Every sniffle, every fever is a battle won, a reminder of the body's resilience in the face of adversity. In the intricate ballet of homeostasis, the body maintains equilibrium amid the ever-changing landscape. From temperature regulation to hormonal balance, the body orchestrates a delicate balancing act. It is a reminder that, even

in the face of chaos, the body is wired to restore balance and preserve its internal sanctity.

2. The Mind-Body Symbiosis—Harnessing the Power of Thoughts: Our thoughts are not mere whispers in the wind; they hold the potential to shape our reality. The field of psychoneuroimmunology reveals the profound connection between thoughts, the nervous system, and the immune response. Positive thoughts become a beacon of hope, lighting the path to recovery and resilience. Enter the realm of the placebo effect, a testament to the mind's extraordinary healing potential. Belief, a force intangible yet potent, can pave the way for recovery. It is a reminder that the mind, when harnessed with positivity and conviction, can propel the body toward healing, even in the absence of conventional interventions. Amid the chaos of modern life, mindfulness emerges as a beacon of serenity. Practices like meditation and mindful awareness empower individuals to navigate the storms within. By cultivating a conscious presence, one can harness the mind's healing energy, fostering a mental terrain that is fertile for rejuvenation.

3. The Soulful Symphony: Ancient healing traditions across cultures echo a common refrain—the interconnectedness of mind, body,

and spirit. Systems like Ayurveda, Traditional Chinese Medicine, and indigenous healing practices view health as a holistic state, where spiritual well-being intertwines with physical vitality. These traditions beckon us to reconnect with the ancient wisdom that resides within. Venture into nature, and you step into a realm where the spirit finds solace. Scientific studies affirm the therapeutic benefits of nature, from reducing stress to enhancing overall well-being. Nature's embrace serves as a reminder that the spirit finds renewal in the simplicity of the natural world, rekindling the flame within. In the pursuit of holistic healing, the spirit finds sustenance in a sense of purpose. A life imbued with meaning becomes a source of inspiration and resilience. Purpose propels us forward, infusing each step with intention and reminding us that healing is not merely a physical journey but a profound odyssey of the spirit.

From my experience working with patients, one of my most profound observations is how negative thinking can significantly impact both the physical body and spirit. The mind-body connection is powerful, and pessimistic thoughts can manifest physically, leading to increased stress levels, weakened immune function, and heightened susceptibility to various health issues. Chronic negativity is often associated with chronic illness and elevated cortisol levels, which can contribute to inflammation and disrupt the body's natural balance. Moreover, the spirit, or one's emotional and mental well-being, can be profoundly affected by harmful thinking. It can lead to feelings of despair, anxiety, and a diminished sense of purpose. Cultivating a positive mindset is not only beneficial for mental health but also contributes to overall physical well-being, promoting resilience and a more harmonious connection between the mind, body, and spirit.

WHY DO YOU THINK IT'S SO IMPORTANT FOR PEOPLE TO BE AWARE OF HOW THE BODY HEALS ITSELF?

As I get older, one of the things that seems to stand out is the importance of listening to our bodies and cultivating intuitive knowledge we have within and using that as a vital tool to maintaining overall well-being. Our bodies possess a remarkable ability to communicate their needs and signals, often manifesting through sensations, emotions, and subtle cues. Tuning into these signals allows us to understand when rest is required, when stress levels are elevated, or when nourishment is needed. Intuitive knowledge within, often referred to as gut feelings or instincts, can guide us in making decisions that align with our physical and emotional needs. Whether it's recognizing the importance of self-care, adjusting our lifestyle, or responding to stressors, developing an awareness of our body's messages and trusting our intuitive knowledge fosters a harmonious connection between mind, body, and spirit. This mindful approach to self-awareness enhances our ability to navigate life's challenges and promotes a holistic sense of health and balance.

Healing, at its essence, is fundamental to the human experience, as it allows us to journey toward becoming whole—a process of mending and reassembling the broken or damaged fragments within oneself. It involves the restoration of a sense of completeness, enabling an individual to feel good once more and cultivate greater resilience for the future. While healing frequently entails enduring moments of discomfort and pain, it is through this transformative process that individuals gain profound insights into themselves. The journey of healing is, in essence, an exploration of self-discovery, illuminating the aspects of oneself that require attention and nurturing for overall well-being and flourishing.

As we navigate the labyrinth of life, the journey of holistic healing beckons—a journey that transcends the physical and delves into the realms of mind, body, and spirit. The body's ability to heal itself from the inside out is not a passive process but an active collaboration between the resilient physical body, the transformative power of the mind, and the ever-nurturing spirit. In embracing this narrative of self-healing, we find not only motivation but a profound invitation to unlock the latent potential within, embarking on a transformative odyssey toward holistic wellness. The power to heal resides within; it is time to unlock the door and step into the radiant realm of self-discovery and renewal.

WHAT ADVICE DO YOU HAVE FOR CREATING HEALTH AND VITALITY FROM THE INSIDE OUT?

In a world saturated with information offering insights on achieving a healthy, energetic, and symptom-free life, navigating through the sea of trendy products and health fads can be both disorienting and seemingly insurmountable. Amid this overload, I propose a simple yet powerful strategy: You are the architect and creator of your own life; you possess the ability to evaluate, remove, and integrate a multitude of practices and habits that collectively contribute to the establishment of robust and enduring health. By focusing on building wellness from the ground up, you construct a resilient house of health that withstands the test of time. This approach also grants an invaluable understanding of the intricacies of your unique needs and desires in the realm of health. Embark on a journey of exploration through nourishment, movement, breathing, setting personal boundaries, creating healthy connections, and living a life of purpose. While universal truths exist in the realm of health, it is crucial to recognize you have the autonomy to tailor these habits to align with the distinctive contours of your own life. Embrace this autonomy as you shape your path to holistic well-being.

About the Author

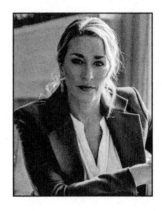

Bethany Miller is a registered nurse and the owner and founder of Aroga Home Care Services. With an unwavering commitment to senior care, Bethany and her company are dedicated to a holistic and high-quality approach to elderly care, considering the complete well-being of individuals — addressing their physical, emotional, and spiritual needs. Bethany resides on the shores of Lake Wylie in South Carolina. She shares her life with her soul partner, her three biological children, and her two bonus children.

Her journey took a unique turn as a young mother when her eldest son, born autistic and blind, became her greatest teacher. She believes those chosen to care for special children are handpicked by The Divine to experience the profound contrasts of life — embracing both its challenges and blessings. In her South Carolina home, Bethany has manifested her dream of creating a sanctuary—a safe haven for her blended family and friends to authentically express themselves. For the children, it serves as an informal university, guiding them through life's intricacies and fostering the development of character and the true meaning of love. Bethany finds joy in crafting beautiful spaces and, through her life's work, continues to contribute positively to the lives of seniors and her extended family.

"I encourage you to embark on a journey of self-discovery, embracing practices of gratitude and resilience. Nurture your physical, spiritual, and emotional well-being to unlock your full potential. I invite you to connect with me and share the details of your journey, where your story is not just heard but celebrated, as you realize the incredible strength you have within."

Bethanylmiller@gmail.com

Bradley Nelson

WHEN AND HOW DID YOU FIRST DISCOVER THAT THE BODY HAS THE INNATE ABILITY TO HEAL ITSELF?

When I was thirteen years old, I was diagnosed with a potentially fatal kidney disease. Western medicine had no treatment available. If my kidneys failed, there was no option of receiving a kidney transplant because the technology was not available at that time. My parents made it possible for me to receive treatments from some holistic doctors who began treating me through spinal realignment, which had an undeniable and immediate effect on me. The severe and intermittent pains I had been suffering immediately reduced in both severity and frequency, and within a few weeks I was feeling completely well.

My parents took me back to the original medical clinic, where I was found to be disease-free. Although the medical profession was able to diagnose me and pronounce me well, they had done absolutely nothing to help me recover. It was then I realized the power to heal the body lies within the body itself. If conditions can be made right, if the blockages that are in the way of healing can be removed, healing can occur without any outside interference. My experiences with patients over thirty-five years as a natural healer have confirmed this to me countless times.

WHY DO YOU THINK IT'S SO IMPORTANT FOR PEOPLE TO BE AWARE OF HOW THE BODY HEALS ITSELF?

It's crucial for people to understand the divine nature of these bodies of ours, and that they are capable of healing themselves. Otherwise, they remain in danger of being at the mercy of corporations whose primary interest is profit. Healthcare, or "Sickness Care," is an enormously profitable business. Pharmaceutical companies don't make any money from a population healthy and taking care of its own needs. Instead, we are conditioned to believe Western medicine has all the answers. We are conditioned to believe if we have physical pain, we need some kind of pharmaceutical drug. We grow up seeing countless ads on television telling us no matter what problem we may have, there is a drug that can cure it. In the West, we are the most conditioned, the most propagandized culture that has ever existed. Part of my job as a teacher is to help create the cognitive dissonance that arises for people when they begin to wake up and realize the incredible power within their own bodies to heal themselves in nearly all circumstances. There will always be a need for Western medicine, but the vast majority of time most people don't need drugs or surgery. They just need to find and remove the blockages in the way of their ability to heal.

WHAT ADVICE DO YOU HAVE FOR CREATING HEALTH AND VITALITY FROM THE INSIDE OUT?

In order to answer this question, let me first discuss the obvious. It's important to consume organic food when possible, and as little processed food as you can. It's important to get enough sleep, to think positive thoughts, to drink plenty of water, to take vitamins and minerals on a regular basis, to get regular exercise, and so on.

What is less obvious is the idea there can be other, unknown problems Western medicine is, for the most part, unaware of.

For example, trapped emotions, or the emotional energies that become lodged in the body during the highs and lows of our lives, are an enormous source of physical pain, as well as the most significant underlying cause of depression, anxiety, panic attacks, phobias, PTSD, eating disorders, self-sabotage, and more. Over thirty-five years of practice, I have found these emotional energies to be a contributing factor in every disease my patients were suffering from.

There are other imbalances that cause us to lose our health and our ability to recover. Many of these exist only on the quantum level and are invisible and completely unrecognized by Western medicine, yet they are taking a tremendous toll on the health of mankind. Still other imbalances have to do with low-grade infection, nutritional deficiencies, toxins of all sorts, misalignments of body tissues, and subtle imbalances of organs, glands, meridians, and more.

It's been my life's work to bring transparency to the human body and its inner workings. The two books that I have written, *The Emotion Code* and *The Body Code*, are my contributions to an awakening world. To me, there's nothing more exciting than seeing the proverbial scales fall from people's eyes as they suddenly realize the vast power that lies within them to recover from illness without drugs or surgery and to be truly healthy and happy by removing the imbalances that lie within.

About the Author

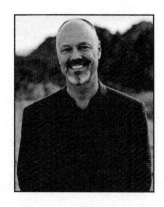

Dr. Bradley Nelson (D.C., ret.) has emerged as a global pioneer in the realm of energy medicine, with a particular emphasis on emotional well-being and holistic health. His groundbreaking methodologies, The Emotion Code and The Body Code, alongside the newly introduced Belief Code, have set new standards in energy healing. As the creator of these innovative systems and the CEO of Discover Healing, Dr. Nelson has cultivated a holistic education platform that not only trains but also certifies practitioners across the globe, equipping them with the tools to unlock the body's inherent ability to heal itself at DiscoverHealing.com.

The impact of Dr. Nelson's work extends far beyond the traditional confines of medicine. His best-selling book, The Emotion Code, now available in an updated and expanded edition, has sold more than half a million copies worldwide and ignited an international energy healing movement. This book provides readers with a profound understanding of how to release trapped emotions, which Dr. Nelson identifies as a core cause of physical and emotional imbalance. His teachings have been validated by the success of over 12,000 certified practitioners who employ his techniques to foster healing and wellness. The addition of a new chapter on inherited emotions, among other enhancements in the latest edition of *The Emotion Code*, further demonstrates Dr. Nelson's commitment to deepening our understanding of holistic health and the power of energy medicine.

Learn more at Discover Healing.com and www.EmotionCodeGift.com

Kerstin Opitz

WHEN AND HOW DID YOU FIRST DISCOVER THAT THE BODY HAS THE INNATE ABILITY TO HEAL ITSELF?

That process happened over time. The very first time, I was nine or ten years old and my mom had a really bad migraine. Her best friend was there, and she showed us how to do acupressure on my mom's feet. Obviously, I was completely clueless as a kid, but as I did it, my mom said she could feel the migraine flow right out of her. That was the "wait a minute" moment.

When I was eleven, I fell off a horse (and was not going to admit it), so I jumped right back on, but I had jammed my hip with that fall. I could barely walk right after it happened. We had a neighbor who was a chiropractor. I had no idea what that meant but when his wife heard what happened, she said, "Bring her over; he'll take a look at her," and that was my first chiropractic adjustment. With that adjustment, I was pain-free. I could walk, no problem.

That was a moment of "What just happened here?" This did not take anything aside from somebody just supporting my body, helping things get back in alignment.

The final push, though, happened when I had fibromyalgia. It started when I was eleven or twelve years old and lasted for thirteen years. We went to the medical doctors first, and they didn't help. It thoroughly went away in grad school when I adjusted my nutrition, my sleep, and my supplementation. All of those pieces brought me back to health. All the medical stuff they threw at me—and some of the tests were really painful—none of that helped me at all. But all the natural healthy things that supported me got me back to health.

Now all of the things I do for myself, my family, and my patients are all natural—all working with the body because that is truly the only thing which ever helped me or my family. It has been absolutely amazing.

WHY DO YOU THINK IT'S SO IMPORTANT FOR PEOPLE TO BE AWARE OF HOW THE BODY HEALS ITSELF?

When I truly learned the body can heal itself, it changed my life, my family's life, and my patients' lives. When we take a medication, it just covers the symptom and usually causes other side effects. We are not healing the body with it; we are not actually supporting it. The symptom is always there to tell us when something is going on—something we would not know without the symptom.

We all have our health paradigm. It is a very broad range, all the way from "The body is dumb, and we have to slice and dice and stuff all of these toxins into it to function, because, otherwise, the body could not do a thing" to "The body knows how to heal itself and all we have to do is support that or remove the interference."

I am very much on "the body heals itself" side, and we just have to remove the interference. I'm also very thankful for the medical side in case of emergency. I always joke with my patients—if you get into an accident and your arm is dangling off, let them sew it on first, and then we can heal you after that.

It really is about figuring out where you stand on the paradigm because that is going to guide your approach to healing. To me, it's about working with your body, and your body is never against you. It felt like my body was against me when I had fibromyalgia until I learned my body was trying to tell me what was wrong. The message is not always clear; we have to figure out what it means. Once we do, we can heal. For me, that meant I did not have debilitating pain. I did not have the mental fog anymore. I did not have the leg stiffness. All of that stuff is gone. Because the issue, the actual cause of it, is gone.

It really is about working with your body and learning how the body can heal itself. Learning that changes everything because I actually get to live my life. I do not have to worry about being debilitated by pain again. I can live my life and do the things I love. I want that for everyone.

WHAT ADVICE DO YOU HAVE FOR CREATING HEALTH AND VITALITY FROM THE INSIDE OUT?

There are a few things to get started, and they are all interconnected. Toxicities are a big topic I work on with all of my patients. Our world has been made to be pretty toxic, with toxic chemicals, heavy metals, EMFs (which are making the mold issue worse), and parasites. These toxins can cause everything from weight gain to attention issues, period problems to brain issues, and so much more.

We need to learn where we are exposed to toxins because the number one step is reducing toxic exposures as best as we can. We need to support the body—the organs and fluids—along with resolving nutrient deficiencies, so we can get to a level where we can safely do a detox. It doesn't do anyone any good to just randomly do a detox; normally, that leads to redistributing toxins in the body and feeling like crap.

The simplest starting point for this is making sure you get good sleep every night, cutting out sugar and processed food, drinking filtered water, moving your body daily, and getting outside. There are many more free tools and specifics beyond this on my website.

Here is a really important aspect usually overlooked or flat-out shoved aside: You need to take care of yourself from a place of love. What I mean is, do all of those healthy things for yourself because you want to take care of yourself, because you want to be healthy. The opposite of this is coming from a place of fear. Typically that's where people want to beat the disease, are fighting the disease . . . are basically turning their body into a battleground, and you can't win health from there. That thinking comes from Western medicine, but remember the body is always on your side. All the symptoms we experience are the body telling us what is going on, so we need to work with the body.

Dealing with health problems can feel really scary and intimidating. There are tools to help overcome that and move back into a space of love. My favorite tool for this is EFT, Emotional Freedom Techniques, sometimes called *Tapping*. It allows you to feel all your emotional heavy stuff and work through it, while also changing your brain pattern and lowering cortisol levels. It's really easy to use, and you can easily use it in the moment. I teach it to a lot of my patients and do sessions with those who have more in-depth issues.

All of that is to say, healing is possible. I see it as: what the body created, the body can heal. We just have to create the right environment to allow for that.

About the Author

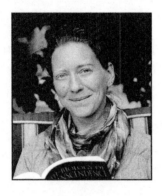

Dr. Kerstin Opitz, originally from Germany, earned her Doctor of Chiropractic at Life University in Marietta, GA. She has been helping patients for over a decade with her unlimited healthy, whole-body approach to her patients' healing. After her own health struggles that started at eleven years old and went undiagnosed for years, her healing journey inspired her to further specialize in nutrition, toxicities, and Emotional Freedom Techniques (EFT). Her passion for supporting the health of her patients led her to become a Certified by the Academy Council of Chiropractic Pediatrics (CACCP) practitioner, caring for pregnant women and newborns. Rooted in her deep appreciation for all the human body is capable of, she has an innate ability to meet people where they are on their own health journey. Guiding her patients at their own pace to heal and achieve their health goals is her great joy. Health is a journey. Rather than focusing on what we cannot control, Dr. K seeks to emphasize the many facets that guide our bodies to their optimal health.

If you're curious to learn more, check out Dr. K's website for courses and free articles here: unlimitedhealthy.com

John Stringer

WHEN AND HOW DID YOU FIRST DISCOVER THAT THE BODY HAS THE INNATE ABILITY TO HEAL ITSELF?

My first encounter was my first injury as a child when I watched how quickly my body responded and healed itself. As I aged, I watched that response shift over time. I began to have other encounters, other challenges that showed me something was shifting, and I eventually sought help.

I received help when I had food, dairy, and several other types of allergies. I was down to five items I could eat that didn't cause a reaction. I received a message in meditation—go to a practitioner, whom someone recommended—the wonderful Doctor Mark Armstrong, in Atlanta, Georgia. He was able to help my body heal itself in a way that was unexpected. In twenty-four hours, I released the food allergies, sugar reactions, and candida; all of those things gone. No more reactions.

When I went back to him, he helped me deal with the final thing I had not told him about lactose intolerance in a single visit. He used multiple modalities, and my body released it all. That showed me my inner knowing is aware of what I need to do to assist my body in healing itself. It also introduced me to many magnificent ways and modalities that can support our bodies in healing themselves.

WHY DO YOU THINK IT'S SO IMPORTANT FOR PEOPLE TO BE AWARE OF HOW THE BODY HEALS ITSELF?

It is important for people to be aware of how the body heals itself so they can work with their innate power and find the practices and modalities that work best for them. Even in working with other modalities outside of that wonderful doctor, I began to learn what my body benefits from and tried other things like Emotional Freedom Techniques (EFT), supplements, redox molecules, and all sorts of vitamins. I began to see other benefits and watched my body respond with mental clarity and energy. I learned what supports my body, my blood type, what my blood type needs and thrives on, my unique expression, and what I seem to be most energized by. Understanding this helps my body function at its best and reduces inflammation. All the practices I have been using and benefiting from come from the knowledge of, "Wow, if I give my body what it needs, it can do the work. It can do the healing."

It's similar to finding practices that work for us in our spiritual development. It is the same; they are connected. Finding those things—our relationship with our food, relationship with our emotions, relationship with our physicality—and bringing them together in harmony helps us achieve alignment with our soul's blueprint. That combination may look different from person to person, but it is our journey to find what works for us. That's where the blessings come in. Even the journey of searching and discovering, in and of itself, is a blessing.

WHAT ADVICE DO YOU HAVE FOR CREATING HEALTH AND VITALITY FROM THE INSIDE OUT?

Find the practices that work for you. Find a framework that brings alignment from the physical, the emotional, and the relationship with your higher power—the divine intelligence you can call the spiritual. Find a balance and create the practices to touch all of those.

When you relate to your body, you are relating to your energy, vibration, and frequencies that compose them and really relating to the innate intelligence that has created it. At the source is a powerful, loving intelligence—a oneness helps and guides us. If you listen to it, it directs you how to bring your life into alignment in all the other areas. Start there as the foundation and cultivate those practices. Then, it will help you know what to give your body and will bring you into the right relationship with other physical appearances.

By cultivating those practices, your body will function more efficiently, and you will begin to attract things to support your expression of physicality. When you create more harmony in your life, you are able to support others and flow in a wonderful giving and receiving.

Find a right relationship with nature — find the part of your harmony as physicality and realize we are all expressions of nature — beings connected with nature. Find your rhythm in rituals and practices to bring you in harmony with that wonderful consciousness, with those vibrations, and with the gifts nature brings us which help us thrive and heal as well.

About the Author

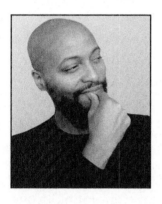

John Stringer is a life teacher, speaker, Billboard-charting singer-songwriter, healer, and author with a passion for music, community, expansion, and limitless love and light. A graduate of Morehouse College, he serves as Founder of PolyPlat Records and ConsciousSongwriting.com. He is a Partner at Healing Arts Management and ConsciousSongwritingRetreat. com. He is co-host of the *Awakened Pillow Talk* podcast with his wife, Kathy, and host of *The Alignment Podcast*.

John has written and recorded numerous singles and albums over the years, including a co-written Billboard Top 10 hit with his former rock band, State of Man. He speaks and sings for events and venues throughout the world, including those he co-produces at Healing Arts Management.

He shares a message of alignment with Source/God through songs on his debut solo album, *Limitless Love & Light*—featuring the Posi Award-nominated songs "That's Love," "You Are Welcome Here," and the spoken word offering, "Power of Love" and "#blacklivesmatter;" his follow-up album, *Moment to Moment (Live)*; and through sharing inspired teachings, some found in his book, *The Abundance Vibration: A Guide to Alignment*. Visit johnstringerinc.com for more information.

Download your digital copy of the *Align. Allow. Let Go.* meditations album from John Stringer FREE, featuring spiritual technology in the form of guided meditations that assist you in aligning with Source/God/Spirit/Genius from moment to moment and accessing genius/guidance from Source.

Step 1: Visit https://bit.ly/jsi-medalbum

Step 2: Use the following Coupon Code upon checkout: TIE2MEDITATION

Ishita Todi

WHEN AND HOW DID YOU FIRST DISCOVER THAT THE BODY HAS THE INNATE ABILITY TO HEAL ITSELF?

When I was about five or six years old, as my mother and I were walking home, I tripped and fell on the ground. I cut my knee and it was bleeding, but I didn't see it. I got up, brushed off my hands, and continued walking. We reached home in a few minutes, as we were just around the corner when I fell. I saw the blood on reaching home, and it had trickled down my shin. And then it all began. I started crying. It started paining. I thought I was going to die. That day was life-changing, but I didn't know it then. My mother and grandfather soothed me; they cleaned the cut, and we had a talk. I had walked from the corner of the road all the way home without feeling the pain, simply because I hadn't seen it. They told me that it was blood. Blood runs through our entire body and keeps us alive. But we don't see it every day and, somehow, as soon as we see it—maybe it's the colour red, or thoughts associated with it—something is triggered in us. It's a sense of *Something is not right. This shouldn't be here.* That one conversation and one incident were the beginning. They laid the foundation for my core beliefs about the body. These beliefs are valid in other contexts as well.

1. Everything is fine in its place. It becomes a problem when it's misplaced.

2. What we don't know doesn't hurt us.

3. The body knows how to heal itself. Let it.

And, as for that cut, it was cleaned, some antiseptic was applied, and it was closely observed and discussed in the following days. First it dried up; then the body quickly formed a little scab to protect itself. As the skin beneath repaired itself, the scab was gently pushed upwards and, finally, the scab was shed by the body. The new skin forming was itchy, drawing my attention to the exact location and reminding me to clean and moisturise it. That was my body's way of telling me to take care of it. As the skin formed and the body repaired itself, it no longer felt the need to send this message. The scar, however, remained for a while longer — another reminder something had happened there, this time as a caution to be careful.

As more time passed, even the scar healed, and I forgot about the fall. Years later, I asked myself this question: *When did I first discover the body has the innate ability to heal itself?* This memory flashed across my mind in reply!

I consider myself blessed to have been raised by wise and loving parents and a patient and generous grandfather. It does take a village to raise a child, and my village had uncles and aunts who were passionate about showing me the world through their experiences.

WHY DO YOU THINK IT'S SO IMPORTANT FOR PEOPLE TO BE AWARE OF HOW THE BODY HEALS ITSELF?

Deep down, people know their body is capable of healing itself and it does heal itself. They've just forgotten. They need to be reminded. They need to remember who they really are, what they're capable of, and why they're living this life.

We all do the same things: eating, sleeping, working, talking, and singing, to name just a few. And yet, the way we do them is different because we are all unique. Each one of us has travelled our individual unique journeys to be here at this point in time. The way our body heals itself is also unique, even though we all follow the same steps. We all have our own individual unique way of connecting and communicating with our bodies, of recognising what is to be done.

Some actions, practices, habits, and patterns need to be reduced and ideally eliminated, while some need to be increased, with new ones introduced, so the body can heal itself. We need to change how we're living so we reduce harming and exhausting, dis-balancing, and dis-harmonising our bodies. We need to work towards a state of being where we require less healing. Our body restores itself when we rest, and we just need to know when and how to rest it.

There is immense empowerment in achieving this state, and empowerment is the only way, the only path to peace. As more people realise their potential power inside their bodies to be a certain way, to feel a certain way, to function in a certain way, the empowerment paves the way for peace. Peace in our homes, in our relationships, in our communities, in our societies, in our countries, and in the world.

WHAT ADVICE DO YOU HAVE FOR CREATING HEALTH AND VITALITY FROM THE INSIDE OUT?

I ask my clients to think of their body as their home. Home is a physical space we live in. Unlike our home, which we might share with others, our body is exclusively our own.

If you were to repair, clean, or decorate your home, how would you go about it?

It has to begin with identification, not just of the area you want to work on, but also what you want to achieve. In the same way, when we work on the body, we start with identification of the location and the desired outcome.

Next, remove some items and create space for the changes. In the body, we need to remove the unwanted energy to create space for the new. The location and energy being removed will require their own treatment just as in your home. Some items can be simply thrown in the trashcan, while some need heavy lifting to be carried out.

After this, carefully choose how you want to rearrange your home and what you want to add. Similarly, in the body, we think carefully about what energy we want to bring in. We use memories and imagination to procure the energy we want.

Once the new arrangement is in place, it takes some getting used to at home. Likewise, our body needs some time to absorb the new energy comfortably.

Finally, there's excitement, joy, satisfaction, and even a feeling of celebration after we complete the renovation at home. In exactly the same way, our body also needs a celebration to complete the exercise of healing.

And no matter how many trends we follow, our home can never be identical to another, simply because we are all unique. Our bodies and our understanding of ourselves can also never be identical for the same reason. We may learn the same healing modality — and yet our practice of it will be different from others. We may follow the same diet as someone else and our bodies will respond differently. Today, there are many people sharing stories of their healing journeys. We can take as long as we need to find the ones we resonate with the most and create our own version for ourselves.

In the beginning, everyone needs a guide, and it's important to choose someone who uplifts you and builds your confidence. Once you're on your journey, you will learn to trust your instincts and listen to your body. Your body is your best guide. It has all the wisdom you will ever need. All you really need is to learn how to communicate with it and all communication is built on good listening. The more you listen to it, the more your body will talk to you. You will then be able to tell your body what you want it to do for you.

About the Author

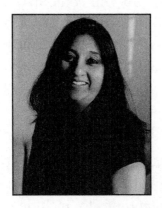

I am an Awakened Parent, and I invite you to join me on this journey. We're all parenting someone or something constantly — our children, homes, businesses, siblings, friends, pets, neighbors, and even our parents — often neglecting our inner child, who needs us the most!

I have been meditating for thirty years and working with energy healing for eighteen years. I have gathered experience through my personal life situations as well as my clients' journeys.

I have been married to my high school sweetheart for twenty-five years, and we have three beautiful children we are very proud of. They are testimony to my methods.

I am happy to share my stories with whomever they might inspire.

On this journey, you will come to a phase when you want to retreat into yourself. Do not be afraid, for this is your time to work on yourself. Just like a butterfly, when you emerge from this phase, you will be ready to spread your wings and fly — not afraid to show yourself to the world. You will carry your own healing story to share with anyone who needs it.

Awakened Parenting brings you specially curated programs designed to enable a conscious expansion in your understanding to include every aspect of your life — physical, financial, emotional, mental, and spiritual.

Write to me at ishita@anawakenedparent.com, and I'll send you a form. The information you provide will help me offer you relevant programs.

Amandha D. Vollmer

WHEN AND HOW DID YOU FIRST DISCOVER THAT THE BODY HAS THE INNATE ABILITY TO HEAL ITSELF?

From my earliest recollections as a child, the inherent capacity of the body to self-heal was an intuitive understanding, as natural and unquestionable as the cycles of the seasons. It was evident in the response of my own body to the myriad small injuries of childhood — the bumps, bruises, cuts, bites, and stings. Each incident served as a testament to the remarkable ability of the body to initiate its own repair — a process that unfolded seamlessly and autonomously.

However, in the unfolding of modern life, these inherent truths of our natural world are systematically overshadowed and replaced. Children, entrusted with the wisdom of their own bodies and the natural world, are gently guided away from this intrinsic knowledge. Instead, societal norms dictate reliance on external authorities and institutions, emphasizing the need for doctors to ensure wellness and schools to impart wisdom.

This departure from nature's innate wisdom becomes a generational betrayal, perpetuating the belief the natural world is fraught with peril and mystery, accessible only through the lens of academic qualification. In my own childhood, amid the whispering leaves of the trees, I inherently grasped their connection to the elements, their seasonal rhythms, and their ability to create medicine for self-healing. These profound insights, unfiltered by external influence, provided a profound understanding of our innate self-healing capabilities, intricately woven into the fabric of the natural world.

However, personal experiences, marked by early medical interventions and the ensuing consequences, revealed the limitations and often detrimental effects of conventional medical approaches. The infliction of pasteurized cow milk instead of the nourishing embrace of maternal milk initiated a trajectory of pain from infancy, a trajectory accentuated by the arrogant ignorance of medical professionals. It became a journey marked by the realization that doctors, despite their authority, often exacerbated rather than alleviated suffering.

As the passage of time unfolded, the tragic decline of my grandparents under the care of these same medical practitioners further underscored the inherent flaws in conventional treatments. Simultaneously, my exploration into herbal and energy medicine revealed the potential for healing beyond the confines of conventional practices. It became increasingly clear, by allowing the body to function without interference, providing essential building blocks for repair, and respecting its innate wisdom, a path of self-resolution emerges.

In the realization that the synthetic world disrupts the harmonious balance of nature while the natural world fosters connection and correction, a profound paradigm shift occurred. The teachings evolved into a guiding principle: for healing, we must offer the body the nourishment it requires, facilitate the elimination of waste, and discern areas of stagnation or blockages — the loci of mistakes, lessons, and gifts inherent in each experience.

The understanding deepened. Challenges in life are not arbitrary but purposeful, a part of nature's design intended for growth and expansion rather than mere existence. As we navigate these challenges, we unfold our inherent potential for resilience, growth, and profound interconnectedness with the natural world from which our healing springs forth.

WHY DO YOU THINK IT'S SO IMPORTANT FOR PEOPLE TO BE AWARE OF HOW THE BODY HEALS ITSELF?

In the absence of awareness, one finds oneself subjected to the capricious whims of chance, disconnected from the intrinsic knowledge that empowers the self. It is an unfortunate surrender of personal authority to illusory figures and institutional doctrines. The resulting vibrational resonance is one of fear, a stark departure from the harmonious frequencies of love and interconnectedness.

As beings of energy and electricity, our thoughts emanate energy fields, our hearts project unique vibrations, and our physical presence influences the resonance with the world around us. These dynamic forces, shaped by our awareness or lack thereof, dictate the nature of our experiences and the energies we attract. In the absence of conscious awareness, a state of spiritual disorientation prevails, leading to a profound disconnect and ailing of the soul.

To be adrift in confusion, swayed by random suggestions and ensnared in the web of collective hypnosis, is to forfeit spiritual bearings. The consequence is a malaise of the soul, a forgetfulness of inherent power, connection to the Source, and the preciousness of life's finite existence. In this disconnection, the natural governance of our being is relinquished, paving the way for the insidious infiltration of addictive tendencies, indecision, fear, and a persistent dwelling in the lower realms of emotional experience.

Yet, when the awareness of our profound connection is reinstated, when the understanding of our unique essence unfolds, and the realization dawns that support and love are perennial companions, a transformative shift occurs. In this awakening, the inherent design for healing, growth, and accomplishment becomes evident, imparting purpose, direction, and clarity to our journey. Without this foundational awareness, vulnerability prevails, rendering us susceptible to manipulation, control, and transformation into empty vessels devoid of a spiritual compass. The importance of understanding how the body heals itself lies in its capacity to restore not only physical well-being but also to reclaim spiritual sovereignty, fostering resilience, purpose, and an unwavering connection to the essence of life itself.

WHAT ADVICE DO YOU HAVE FOR CREATING HEALTH AND VITALITY FROM THE INSIDE OUT?

To cultivate health and vitality from the inside out, embark on a journey of self-reflection and introspection. Pause amid the whirlwind of life, engaging in a conscious act of taking stock. Cease all action, look within, and listen intently to the inner voice that often whispers amid the clamor of external noise. In this stillness, amplify the volume of your inner wisdom, tuning into its nuanced guidance.

Allow yourself the gift of solitude, free from distractions, immersing in the depth of your feelings with unyielding bravery. Confront and release bodily traumas, recognizing that memories and traumas reside in the physical form. Employ movement, shaking, tapping, and the freedom to cry as conduits for the release and resolution of stored traumas and tensions. It is a process often circumvented by the allure of organized religion, which, instead of empowering individuals, offers illusory crutches to cope with pain and suffering and instills false savior programming.

Rediscover the sanctity of your own body, acknowledging it as the vessel of salvation. The embodiment of the body of Christ lies within your own acceptance of feelings and enlightenment gained through the courageous exploration of pain and existence's shadows. Elevate yourself into Christ Consciousness by unblocking patterns, allowing the anointing oil to ascend the spine, moving through all the energy centers, and lighting up your crown, fostering resonance with the natural world and your spiritual connection to it. This awakening permits the flow of inner wisdom, the blossoming of innate gifts, and the unhindered manifestation of your own true genius.

Examine your patterns, habits, addictions, needs, wants, and desires, delving into the depths of self-awareness. Liberation emerges through this introspective journey, and salvation flows from the conscious application of waters upon the self. Reconnect with the natural world, grounding your body in its elements, feeling the textures of trees, walking barefoot upon the soil, absorbing the nourishment of the sun, and attuning to the rhythmic dance of water against the shore. Recognize that you are an integral part of this interconnected tapestry.

Reframe your actions within the paradigm of love. Scrutinize whether your behaviors are self-loving or self-destructive. Confront the awareness of detrimental habits—alcohol consumption, reliance on coffee, fast-food consumption, stress mismanagement, insufficient sleep, sedentary lifestyles, and unfiltered media exposure. Envision a life infused with love and contemplate the changes required for your own liberation, detached from societal judgments and warped expectations.

Initiate a revolution of the soul, commencing with honesty and self-reparenting. Step away from operating through the lens of a damaged inner child, seizing spiritual maturity through resolute willpower. In this transformative process, one becomes one's own savior, forging a path toward freedom, authenticity, and a profound connection with the essence of their being. Here is where we discover profound meaning, purpose, and truth.

About the Author

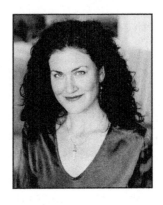

Amandha Dawn Vollmer, affectionately known as ADV, is a renowned health expert and best-selling author with an impressive breadth of knowledge on natural healing and holistic wellness practices. With over twenty years of experience in the field, ADV is a sought-after speaker and educator who has inspired countless individuals to take control of their health and live vibrant, thriving lives. She designs and produces handcrafted and all-natural body care remedies available in her online stores (yumnaturals.store and DMSO.store).

Amandha has also been educating on the scientific errors of the germ theory and teaching a self-empowering method of terrain care. Amandha teaches the truth about this world (gentle or blunt); her breadth of knowledge delves into politics, law, physics, philosophy, corrected history, and cosmology. She has been a voice of sound logic during the plandemic, calling out the hoax on day one, experiencing backlash via violent cancel culture and various harassments, and losing huge social media accounts, etc. She is one of the members of the esteemed Team No-Virus, exposing the fraud of virology and the lies of the germ theory.

Join Amandha's Private Community and participate in specific health-related groups, engage with like-minded holistic healers, educate yourself and others with our step-by-step online courses, access weekly interactive video chats with Amandha, and reach the ultimate natural health lifestyle.

https://yummy.doctor/product/yummy-doctor-memberships

Lisa Warner

WHEN AND HOW DID YOU FIRST DISCOVER THAT THE BODY HAS THE INNATE ABILITY TO HEAL ITSELF?

Throughout my life, I had many sprains, bumps, bruises, and colds, and my body always healed itself from those things. I really discovered the body's ability to heal itself when I found myself facing "cancer." Looking at the medical model's options of chemo, radiation, radical surgery, and/or heavy pharmaceuticals, I did not like any of those options because, to me, they seemed both scary and barbaric. It seemed to me healing should be much simpler, and I knew my body had always healed itself, so why should this be any different?

I decided to get very quiet and inquire inside about what I truly knew about my body, and I asked myself: *If there were no doctors on the planet and I just had to heal myself, what would I do?* My answer was right there, and I decided that I was going to do exactly what my inner guidance told me to do, as if there were no doctors on the planet. I ended up following my own inner guidance, and my body healed itself. It was quite amazing.

WHY DO YOU THINK IT'S SO IMPORTANT FOR PEOPLE TO BE AWARE OF HOW THE BODY HEALS ITSELF?

From my direct experience it is really, really important we all understand how to manage our own bodies because our body is part of us. We are Souls in human form, and we have the full ability to heal ourselves, but we have been programmed to believe somebody else has to do the healing for us.

When I found myself facing "cancer" and decided to heal myself, my inner guidance was able to guide me back to health. I discovered along my journey we are looking at it from a completely backward perspective. We are looking at symptoms that show up in the body, but why did they show up? We are not looking at the energy underneath. We are not looking at what is happening in the mind and the soul.

We cannot separate the body, the mind, and the soul. They have been separated through our society where the doctors have jurisdiction over the body, the religious institutions have jurisdiction over the soul, and the educational system has jurisdiction over the mind. That is how they separate us from the inside out. It is up to us to bring ourselves back together. What I learned with healing my own body is that my mental and emotional state had a direct impact on my physical state. My body was not being attacked by a "disease," but, rather, my body was responding to the emotional and mental input I was giving it. If everybody understood this, we would have little or no need for chemo, radiation, radical surgery, or pharmaceuticals because we each have the ability to bring our own internal compass back into alignment.

WHAT ADVICE DO YOU HAVE FOR CREATING HEALTH AND VITALITY FROM THE INSIDE OUT?

Learn how to be happy. Learn how to allow yourself to feel good no matter what is going on in the external world or with your body. We have been taught that physical sensations and emotions are the same thing. That when our body feels fear, we go into fear and then we justify the fear with thought patterns. *I am afraid because – (fill in the blank)*. What I have learned is that everything is energy. Fear is an energy. Guilt is an energy. Shame is an energy. When those energies are in our energy fields they will play out as our reality.

When we learn how to clear those low-vibe, anti-life energies out of our energy fields, they stop playing out in our reality and we begin to be *happy!* I used to carry a lot of anger, fear, and resentment, which my body eventually displayed as "cancer," at which point I became angry at, resentful of, and afraid of my own body. I then began using my body as the justification for feeling *angry, resentful,* and *afraid.* Once I learned how to clear those energies out of my energy field, I realized there was nothing to *resent, to be angry about,* or to be *afraid of* anymore. Once I stopped fearing my body and learned to *trust* it instead, everything changed. It is really important that people learn how to clear low vibe negative emotions from their energy fields because once we realize that everything is energy, we can start making rapid changes for the better, for ourselves, and for humanity.

About the Author

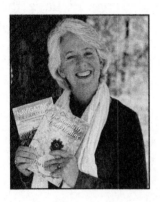

Lisa Warner is an award-winning, international bestselling author of *The Simplicity of Self-Healing*, now in its 10th Anniversary Edition. She wrote the book after healing herself from cancer naturally, without the use of the medical model. During her journey of self-healing, she learned that cancer is *not* the problem that it is made out to be, and is, in fact, the body's *solution* to a problem. It is how the body assists us through times of emotional turmoil. Once she realized there was nothing to fear, she was able to trust her body to heal itself — which, of course it did … naturally, without special diets, pills, or medical protocols of any kind.

Lisa is passionate about showing us who we truly are … Angels in human form, who are a perfect combination of body, mind, and soul divinely designed for disease-free living.

Her core message is we all have the power to heal ourselves and healing the body is literally an inside job.

Lisa is a bright light and a difference-maker who helps her clients transcend disease as they EmBODY their Soul.

Go to: www.ConnectingYoutoYou.com/freegift to receive a FREE Guided Journey, Creating from the non-Physical Self.

Alec Zeck

WHEN AND HOW DID YOU FIRST DISCOVER THAT THE BODY HAS THE INNATE ABILITY TO HEAL ITSELF?

I first discovered the body has the innate ability to heal itself after witnessing my wife reverse autoimmune conditions. She was diagnosed in 2007, and she suffered with them until 2016 when we began a process of tapering her off of the various pharmaceutical drugs. Up until that point she had been under the care of multiple rheumatologists who told her she would always need to be on pharmaceutical products in order to manage her chronic pain. Of course, the first few pharmaceuticals she was prescribed led to side effects that led to more pharmaceuticals and more pharmaceuticals, and then she was on a never-ending cycle of pharmaceutical drugs that suppressed some symptoms and increased other symptoms.

In 2016, we came across the work of Doctor Kelly Brogan and began a process of tapering my wife off all her medications. We adopted a very natural approach to health—eating organic food, focusing on mindfulness, focusing on breathing deeply, spending adequate time in the sun and out in nature, and moving her body. My wife reversed all of her chronic conditions in a matter of four months and had blood work to prove that by no longer listening to these so-called experts, and by adopting this natural approach to health and no longer using any pharmaceuticals, she had reversed all her chronic conditions for the first time in nearly nine years.

After witnessing this I became aware of the body's innate capacity to heal itself. I also became acutely aware of how the allopathic medical system and the pharmaceutical industry working together condition us to believe that our bodies are broken and defective and there is not much we can do about it aside from outsourcing all of our power and capacity for health to them. This perpetuates the problem making our health deteriorate much quicker than it would in most cases.

WHY DO YOU THINK IT'S SO IMPORTANT FOR PEOPLE TO BE AWARE OF HOW THE BODY HEALS ITSELF?

It is important for people to be aware of how the body heals itself because it brings about legitimate healing. The amount of people my wife and I have come across in the last eight years with stories nearly identical to hers is incredible, and it is inspiring beyond words. You can live a much more fruitful life and a much more joyful life when you understand this truth and embody it. It is a much more empowering perspective to understand that you know best for your body, and your body has all that it needs inside of it in order to maintain vibrant health. By adopting a natural approach to health and utilizing the abundant resources God provides us, you can be healthy. That is a beautiful way to approach life.

WHAT ADVICE DO YOU HAVE FOR CREATING HEALTH AND VITALITY FROM THE INSIDE OUT?

One of the most important components that is often overlooked, even in a lot of alternative health circles, is how much emotions, spiritual health, and metaphysical aspects of health play into the physical expression of symptoms or of wellness. The most important thing one can do is learn to resolve their conditioned beliefs about the world and about themselves and understand, even at the deepest level, this idea we are limited, lacking, finite, and will cease to exist at some point is conditioning.

We have only ever experienced experience itself; we have never experienced not living. We buy into the belief that we are limited and lacking and finite when the reality is we are abundant, self-healing, self-regenerating, and eternal. We need to become acutely aware of our thoughts and how our thoughts, in combination with our feelings, lead us to make decisions not best for our health. We need to recognize how thoughts and feelings can bring about symptoms of illness or negative symptoms in the body and then work to resolve those thoughts and feelings. It is important to focus on diet, movement, getting adequate sunlight, and drinking water. The most important components are our emotions, our conditioned beliefs, and our connection to God.

About the Author

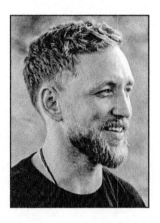

Alec Zeck received his B.S. in Systems Engineering from the United States Military Academy at West Point. He is a speaker, writer, podcaster, and former Army Captain. He is the Founder and former Executive Director of Health Freedom for Humanity, the founder of The Way Forward, and producer of *The End of COVID* series.

https://thewayfwrd.com

https://theendofcovid.com

IG @d_alec_zeck

IG @thewayfwrd

IG @the.way.fwrd (backup account)

Conclusion

Congratulations on reaching the conclusion of this book. It has been our absolute pleasure to introduce you to these inspirational difference-makers we've featured. It is our hope you have learned a lot as you've read and that a world of possibilities has opened up for you. Let this not be a book you read once and put down without taking any action.

We highly suggest reading through this book three times and, with each read, take three action steps toward creating better health and vitality for you, your family, and people you care about.

Which authors did you connect with most?

Which stories really stuck with you?

Who inspired you the most?

Who made you consider exploring new possibilities you may not have considered previously?

Which authors do you feel will support you in your current healing journey?

As a next step, we suggest reaching out to them. Make a connection. See how they may support you moving forward.

We wish you all the best in your healing journey.

About the Publisher

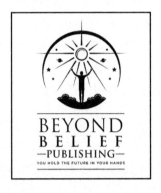

In 2004, Babypie Publishing was founded by entrepreneurs Keith and Maura Leon S. when they decided to self-publish their co-authored book, *The Seven Steps to Successful Relationships*. When Babypie published its second book, Keith Leon's *Who Do You Think You Are? Discover the Purpose of Your Life* a few years later — implementing a large marketing campaign that introduced the book to over a million people on the first day it came out — both books became bestsellers overnight.

After the success of their first two titles, Keith and Maura were approached by another author who believed they could take his book to bestseller status as well. They decided to give it a shot, and Warren Henningsen's book, *If I Can You Can: Insights of an Average Man*, became an international bestseller the day it was released.

Before long, Babypie Publishing was receiving manuscript submissions from all over the world and publishing such titles as Ronny K. Prasad's *Welcome to Your Life*; Melanie Eatherton's *The 7-Minute Mirror*; and Maribel Jimenez and Keith Leon's *The Bake Your Book Program: How to Finish Your Book Fast and Serve It Up HOT!*.

With a vision to make an even greater impact, Babypie Publishing began offering comprehensive writing and publishing programs, as well as a full range of à-la-carte services to support independent authors and innovative professionals in getting their message out in the most powerful and effective manner. In 2015, Keith and Maura developed the YouSpeakIt book program to make it easy, fast, and affordable for busy entrepreneurs and cutting-edge health practitioners to get their mission and message out to the world.

In 2016, Leon Smith Publishing was created as the new home for Babypie, YouSpeakIt, and future projects. In 2018, Beyond Belief Publishing was added as an imprint for spiritual and esoteric titles. They have published well over 100 books.

Whether you're a transformational author looking for writing and publishing services or a visionary leader ready to take your life and work to the next level, we thank you for visiting our website at LeonSmithPublishing. com, and we look forward to serving you.

Printed in Great Britain
by Amazon